# PRINCIPLES OF EFFECTIVE PARENTING

# Also Available

Handbook of Socialization:
Theory and Research, Second Edition
*Edited by Joan E. Grusec and Paul D. Hastings*

# Principles of Effective Parenting

## HOW SOCIALIZATION WORKS

JOAN E. GRUSEC

THE GUILFORD PRESS

New York     London

**Library of Congress Cataloging-in-Publication Data**

Names: Grusec, Joan E., author.
Title: Principles of effective parenting : how socialization works /
  Joan E. Grusec.
Description: New York, NY : Guilford Press, [2019] | Includes
  bibliographical references and index.
Identifiers: LCCN 2019010748 |ISBN 9781462541560 (paperback :
  alk. paper)| ISBN 9781462540396 (hardcover : alk. paper)
Subjects: LCSH: Socialization. | Parenting. | Parent and child.
Classification: LCC HQ783 .G784 2019 | DDC 306.874—dc23
LC record available at *https://lccn.loc.gov/2019010748*

# Preface

There is no more important job in the world than raising the next generation. Children come into the world ready and eager to become part of a social group, but they need guidance and help to learn what the requirements are to be happy and responsible members of that group. They need to learn values and associated behaviors that will assist them in this undertaking. Unfortunately, there seems to be considerable confusion about the best procedures for achieving this learning. Whereas it is relatively easy to follow instructions for baking a cake, driving a car, or building a house, it is not so easy to follow instructions for raising a child. It's not that such instructions do not exist. When I most recently Googled "parenting," I got 286,000,000 hits. "Child rearing" and "childrearing" yielded a total of 6,950,000 hits. The problem is that the rules are often contradictory, even when they are based on research findings. Go along with your children's wishes, but be strict. Respond to your child's crying, but don't, because it will reinforce the undesirable behavior of crying. Spanking in moderation is a useful tool, but it leads to antisocial behavior. Researchers aren't always sure what to conclude from various theories and findings; parents despair of so-called "expert" advice, but they continue to worry about whether they are doing the best job possible.

This book is about the socialization of children—the process by which they learn values and behaviors associated with those values. It focuses primarily on the role parents play in the process. Other individuals and events are also involved in socialization—teachers, peers, grandparents, coaches, siblings, the mass media, and (increasingly) social media—and many of the principles that apply to being a parent are also relevant to these other people and events. But parents have a special role to play for a number of reasons. They are usually assigned the primary role for child rearing; they have to live with their children on a daily basis; and they have a relationship that, unlike other relationships, is extremely difficult to sever.

## ■ THE DOMAIN APPROACH

This book is an attempt to organize existing research in a way that makes it seem less contradictory. This organization has definite implications for practical concerns about raising children. The argument I present is that parenting takes place in different domains, and that the appropriate parenting response depends on the domain in which a child is currently operating. There is no one action that is appropriate across the board. Rather, there are many different ways to achieve the same goal of teaching children how to behave in a socially appropriate way. I suggest that the topics addressed in socialization research can be broken down into five domains, although that does not mean that a different approach to categorization might not yield more domains. Two of the domains provide a foundation for effective learning of values. The remaining three provide different ways of helping children acquire specific values and associated action.

The domains that provide a foundation are "protection" and "reciprocity." Protection involves parents' keeping children safe from danger and helping them cope with upsetting or distressing situations. Children whose parents can be relied upon to be available when comfort and protection are needed feel secure. As a result, they are able to explore their world, confident in the knowledge that they can return to a safe base if life becomes dangerous. Over time, children learn to take on the protection role themselves as they are taught to cope with feelings of distress. When children can cope with their own distress, they also become able to deal with the distress or needs of others. In this way, they adopt behavior that helps them to become better members of the social group. In the protection domain, children also learn to trust their parents to have their best interests at heart, and so they become more willing to go along with parental direction.

The second domain is the reciprocity domain. This is the domain in which parents respond to *reasonable* requests from their children. Such requests frequently occur during play when children want to engage in a particular activity, but they can happen at other times as well. When their wishes are granted, children become more likely to grant their parents' wishes in turn; they are more willing to comply or reciprocate if their parents have built up a store of good will. The reciprocity domain presents a special challenge, as it can require that parents engage in actions they might find boring or time-consuming. But such engagement pays off in the form of children's compliance with parents' requests in future interactions.

The domains that involve teaching children specific values are "control," "guided learning," and "group participation." The control domain is activated when children misbehave and when parents need to respond in some way that will reduce the chances of the misbehavior's recurring. It is a domain in which parents have a particular interest, because a child's misdeeds require an immediate response, and because these misdeeds are frequently accompanied by anger and frustration for parents and child alike. Thus it is the domain where the most research has been conducted. What should a parent do when a child has misbehaved? And, of course, what should a parent do when a child has behaved in a particularly exemplary fashion?

The guided learning domain has received much less formal attention in the socialization literature than the control domain has. It is activated not when children have misbehaved, but when an opportunity arises for a lesson to be learned. In this domain, parents read stories to their children that depict the importance of particular values, or they talk with their children about emotions or behaviors. Guided learning also occurs when parents and children reminisce about past experiences. These previous experiences could include children's antisocial behavior or distress, but the time for discipline or comfort is long gone, and so the interaction now becomes an exchange of views about past events. Finally, in the group participation domain, children observe socially acceptable behavior exhibited by others, as well as take part in rituals, routines, and interactions with others. The latter cement their feelings of group belongingness and encourage them to think that the beliefs and values of their own group are a desirable and appropriate guide for action.

The notion of domains of social life and their role in socialization was initially proposed by Bugental and Goodnow (1998) and Bugental

(2000). The argument was that, rather than being prepared to engage in stable response patterns across different social contexts, children require responses that are conditional on particular situations in which they are currently functioning. Accordingly, children and parents use different rules to manage the distinctive problems associated with basic domains of social life. Further elaboration of this position came in Bugental and Grusec (2006) and Grusec and Davidov (2007, 2010).

## ■ ORGANIZATION

This book consists of eight chapters. The first chapter provides an overview of general issues related to socialization. The second is focused on how researchers have addressed the problem of moral development. The chapter deals with only one value (caring for others), albeit a singularly important one and, accordingly, one that has received considerable research attention. Most of that research deals with issues that are not directly focused on socialization. It is useful, however, to see how it relates to and informs an understanding of socialization. The last chapter offers a set of conclusions about the domains-of-socialization approach. Each of the intervening chapters reviews the research on a particular domain in the socialization literature and is a potentially stand-alone presentation of the five different areas of investigation. Chapters 2–7 each also include a discussion of how, historically, researchers have studied the particular topic being addressed in that chapter. It is, at the very least, an informative exercise to see how thinking has changed over time and what forces have been operating to promote those changes in thinking. Setting theoretical disagreements in this historical context helps us to understand how those disagreements came to be and how they might be resolved.

Throughout the book, use is made of narratives collected during my own research. These narratives come from young adults from a wide variety of cultural groups who were asked to describe a time when they had learned an important value or lesson. Analyses of the narratives provide insights into the mechanisms of learning occurring in each domain. Chapters 3–7 also conclude with examples of children's behavior in the different domains; in each chapter, readers are asked to select which of several possible parenting actions, based on research findings reviewed in that chapter, might be most effective for socialization.

This book is intended primarily for an academic audience, as well as for professionals who work with children and parents or other adults. The ultimate hope, of course, is that the ideas presented here might help parents feel more confident about their socialization practices, and there is no reason that this book might not be helpful for them as well.

## ■ ACKNOWLEDGMENTS

I owe a debt of gratitude to many colleagues, among them former students, who have stimulated and contributed to my thinking about socialization processes. Daphne Bugental is one of those colleagues, and I valued our friendship and interactions highly. Jacqueline Goodnow was also a dear friend and a source of considerable intellectual challenge. Maayan Davidov, once my student, has been closely involved in the development of ideas about domains of socialization, and I am exceedingly grateful that we have been able to work so closely together. I single out four other recently or almost recently graduated students: Maria Chaparro, Tanya Danyliuk, Amanda Sherman, and Julia Vinik. Their wish to translate the domains into an educational program for parents has produced many lively and productive evenings of discussion. Finally, numerous other graduate students, including Courtney Braun, as well as a host of undergraduates who have worked in my lab over the years, have all been important contributors to my thinking and writing about parenting and the socialization process.

I sincerely appreciate the continued financial research support over many years that I have received from the Social Science and Humanities Research Council of Canada, as well as involvement in the research by the families whose members have given so generously of their time as they shared their thoughts and feelings about parenting with me and my students. Thanks also to reviewers of the first draft of this book— John Gibbs, Deborah Laible, Jennifer Lansford, Eric Lindsey, Greg Pettit, and Judi Smetana—for their careful reading and thoughtful suggestions for improvement.

To my family—Bob Lockhart and Carolyn Lockhart—my thanks for your support and caring, with special thanks to Bob for his endless willingness to listen to and critique my thinking.

# Contents

# CHAPTER 1

# How Values Are Learned

## *An Introduction*

This book is about "socialization"—about how new members of a group are helped by older members to acquire the values, norms, beliefs, and behaviors necessary to become successful group members. The process has been described by Bugental and Goodnow (1998) as a continuing collaboration between elders and novices, or old hands and newcomers, as the old hands help the new arrivals become part of the social community. The socialization process occurs in many settings, such as starting a new job, immigrating to a new country, becoming a parent, or joining a social club. In this book, I focus on children as the novices and their parents or primary caregivers as the old hands. It is in the family context that children are prepared to enter and become successful members of the larger social community where they will spend the rest of their lives. Although siblings, teachers, friends, group leaders, coaches, characters portrayed in the mass media, and (increasingly) persons encountered through social media also have roles to play in socializing children, parents are of particular importance because they have greater control over their children, as well as longer and more sustained periods of access to them, than any of these other people.

There are a number of reasons for parents' greater access to and control of their children. First of all, human beings have evolved to have a long period of dependency after birth, and so there is considerable time available for parents to teach values and appropriate behavior. As well, in the majority of cultures, parents are assigned primary responsibility for this teaching. Because they spend so much time with their children, parents have the opportunity to develop relationships with them that are essential for successful socialization. They also have time and opportunity to monitor their children's activities and so to develop knowledge of what their children are doing, as well as to become familiar with their children's predispositions—another essential ingredient for effective socialization. And, possibly most important of all, parents have to live in close proximity to their children. Therefore, in order to ensure their own comfort and well-being, most parents want to be surrounded by well-behaved children who follow the norms and requirements of family and societal functioning.

Successful socialization in the family means that children must learn to regulate or temper their emotions, so that they are able to control feelings of anger, frustration, fear, and sadness that interfere with the display of socially acceptable behavior. They must also acquire the standards, attitudes, and values that direct this behavior. In the course of deliberately socializing their children, parents also less intentionally teach other skills, including ways of resolving conflict and of viewing relationships. As well, their parenting has both a direct and an indirect effect on their children's feelings of self-esteem and self-efficacy. Finally, when parenting is problematic, it can give rise not only to antisocial behavior or externalizing problems, but also to internalizing problems such as anxiety and depression.

## ■ THE IMPORTANCE OF PARENTING

Given all that needs to be accomplished during the course of socialization, as well as its importance, it is easily argued that childrearing is the most significant job there is. Indeed, leaving a mark on the next generation, either as a parent or in some other capacity, is central to a sense of satisfaction with one's life. In *The Children of Men,* written in 1992 and set in 2021, the novelist P. D. James describes a world in which it is no longer possible for people to reproduce. As a result, humanity has lost its future. With no children to rear, people cease caring and become depressed. Democracy is abandoned, a dictator rules, and there is no interest in the arts or other activities. Convicted criminals are sent to a penal colony where they are abandoned, and older people are encouraged to commit suicide. This is a world with no children and no future, and it is far from a happy one—simply because investment in future replacements and in the passing on of experience is what gives meaning to existence.

## ■ FEATURES OF THIS BOOK

There are many books, articles, and websites about parenting in general, and specifically about how children and adolescents can be encouraged to become productive contributors to, and happy members of, society. They are of two sorts: those intended for an academic and professional audience, and those intended to offer helpful suggestions to parents on how to raise their children. In both cases, however, there can be a problem when findings from the research are mixed, or when the content of the advice is contradictory. Thus one approach may emphasize sensitive parenting that is responsive to the needs and wishes of the child. Another underlines the importance of setting limits and the utilization of rewards and punishments in promoting acceptable behavior. In the middle is an approach that encourages the setting of limits and the utilization of consequences, but that also encourages responsiveness to the child's wishes. Some writers approve of occasional spanking under specified conditions, and others see spanking as absolutely harmful under all conditions. Parents are advised to use positive reinforcement, but they are also told that positive reinforcement can be counterproductive. Time out is alleged to be an excellent form of discipline, but only if administered properly. Children should be cocooned or protected from unpleasant experiences, or they should be exposed to them and taught how to cope. It is not surprising, then, that people sometimes despair at the confusion surrounding how to carry out the most important job in the world. Nor is it surprising that an exasperated mother wrote the following about "expert parenting advice":

> Keep the room warm, but not too warm.
> Co-sleeping is the best way to get sleep, except that it can kill your baby, so never, ever do it. If your baby doesn't die, you will need to bed-share until college.
> Don't let your baby sleep too long, except when they've been napping too much, then you should wake them. Never wake a sleeping baby.
> Swaddle the baby tightly, but not too tightly.

You should start a routine and keep track of everything. Don't watch the clock. Put them on a schedule.

Put them on their backs to sleep, but don't let them be on their backs too long or they will be developmentally delayed.

This book is an attempt to sort out some of the contradictions and to organize what is currently known about the socialization of children. To do so, I survey research on the various ways in which values and associated behaviors can be acquired, when it is appropriate to use a particular way, and what that way involves or requires. This approach will, I hope, help readers to make sense of what are apparent inconsistencies and offer a way of categorizing or organizing a very large body of knowledge. The framework for organizing the research comes from a "domains-of-socialization" approach, first proposed by Bugental and Goodnow (1998) and Bugental (2000), and elaborated by Bugental and Grusec (2006) and Grusec and Davidov (2010). This approach views socialization as occurring in several different kinds of situations or contexts, with each context involving different kinds of parent–child interactions and different requirements for successful socialization.

## ■ WHAT ARE THE DOMAINS OF SOCIALIZATION?

To anticipate my later, much lengthier descriptions of the socialization domains, I provide a brief summary here. The first two domains ("protection" and "reciprocity") have to do with the development of a relationship with the parent or agent of socialization that supports the teaching of values and associated behavior in the next three domains ("control," "guided learning," and "group participation"). Specifically, the domains involve the following:

1. *Protection.* Parents act as caregivers and providers of comfort when their children are distressed, as well as help them to deal with distress on their own. As a result, children become secure in the knowledge that they will be kept safe and, ultimately, that they have the ability to cope with distress on their own. The ability to cope with their own distress makes it easier for children to provide assistance to others who are distressed.

Here are two scenarios involving children who are in the protection domain.

*Chris (6 years old) is invited to a neighbor's house to see their new dog. Chris hasn't had much experience with dogs, and he says he's afraid and doesn't want to go. His father tries to help him overcome his fear.*

*Janice (12 years old) comes home from school looking very sad and immediately goes to her room. Her mother asks if anything is wrong. Janice says that she has just had a fight with her best friend and is afraid they will never be friends again. Her mother expresses concern.*

2. *Reciprocity.* An exchange or egalitarian relationship is set up, with parent and child mutually interactive and compliant. This domain reflects an inherent tendency to reciprocate favors: When one partner complies with reasonable requests, the other partner is more likely to comply with that individual's future reasonable requests.

Here are two examples in this domain:

*Alan (5 years old) and his mother are waiting in the airport terminal for their boarding call. Mother is texting, and Alan is bored. He asks his mother if they can go and watch some planes taking off. Mother agrees to do so, if they don't go too far. (Later, on the plane, Alan's mother asks him to stop kicking the seat in front of him, and Alan does so immediately.)*

*Stella (8 years old) asks her father, who is watching the news, to play a card game with her. Dad finds this particular card game especially boring. However, he complies. (Later, Dad asks Stella to bring him the newspaper. Stella does so immediately.)*

3. *Control.* Misbehavior is corrected through the use of reward and punishment, combined with reasoning and explanation. In this domain, the relationship is a hierarchical one, and children are required by their parents to learn to regulate or control their own behavior in accord with societal demands and values.

Here are two examples in the control domain:

*Amanda (8 years old) is extremely difficult to get up in the morning. As a result, she makes other people late for work or school. Her parents try to get her to be more considerate of the other family members' needs.*

*Charlie (14 years old) is frustrated because he can't solve a math problem for school. His mother is trying to help him when his*

*younger brother asks if he can borrow Charlie's new baseball bat.
Charlie yells at his brother and tells him to keep his grubby hands off
his (Charlie's) possessions. Charlie's mother tries to get him to better
control his anger.*

4. *Guided learning.* Appropriate action is encouraged through teaching at the child's level of understanding. The goal here is for the child to internalize or take over the parent's way of thinking, including the parent's values.

Examples of guided learning are as follows:

*Tara (8 years old) and her father walk by a homeless man lying in a
doorway. Tara asks her father why he is lying there. Her father begins
a discussion about people who are homeless and in need.*

*Jimmy (5 years old) likes to have his father read him stories at bed-
time. His father especially likes to select stories that involve being
kind to other people or to animals.*

5. *Group participation.* Information about what is acceptable behavior is acquired through watching others and engaging in routines and rituals, as well as in socially approved activities with others. Socialization in this domain takes advantage of the child's desire to be a member of the group and to be similar to other members of the group. It includes learning by observing others, as well as acquiring values and related actions by actually engaging in desirable behavior with others.

Two examples of group participation are these:

*Terry (12 years old) is not as kind and considerate as his parents would
like him to be. They try to provide examples of kind behavior that will
help him to change. For example, Terry and his parents routinely visit
an animal shelter where they spend time walking the dogs.*

*Grace (8 years old) wants to watch TV with her mother. Her mother
suggests they watch a well-reviewed movie about a young woman
with a disability who trains hard and wins a medal at the Paralympics.*

Table 1.1 summarizes each of those domains. It lists the particular kind of parent–child relationship that is elicited in each domain, what the parent needs to do to be an effective agent of socialization, and how parenting works in that domain. In some cases, the parent is reacting to something the child has done; in other cases, the parent is anticipating

**TABLE 1.1. Domains of Socialization, with Type of Parent–Child Relationship, Nature of Required Parenting, and Mechanism Involved in Each Domain**

| Domain | Relationship | Parenting required | Mechanism |
|---|---|---|---|
| Protection | Provider–recipient of care | Alleviate child's distress | Confidence in protection |
| Reciprocity | Exchange | Grant reasonable requests | Innate tendency to reciprocate |
| Control | Hierarchical | Discipline in effective way | Learning of self-control |
| Guided learning | Teacher–student | Scaffold learning | Internalization of teacher's approach |
| Group participation | Members of the same social group | Expose to positive behavior through observation and participation | Sense of social identity |

what the child might do in the future (and either encouraging or discouraging such future action, depending on its acceptability). Specifically, the protection, reciprocity, and control domains all involve an initial action on the child's part—distress, a request, or behavior of either a positive or negative nature. The guided learning and group participation domains involve parents taking the initiative and engaging in teaching or providing models of positive social behavior, as well as providing opportunities for engaging in such behavior.

This book includes five chapters (Chapters 3–7) that are devoted to each of the domains, with the intention that the categorization into domains will help to highlight central features of socialization and to show how effective parenting can be achieved in each domain. Each of these five chapters begins with a brief historical overview of how research in that particular domain came to be conducted, including its theoretical underpinnings and the way in which conceptualizations of that domain have changed over time. In real life, of course, domains do not operate in isolation, and parent and child often find themselves in more than one domain or moving from one domain into another. I defer a discussion of this to Chapter 8, after each domain has been fully described on its own.

Before I move to a discussion of domains, however, there are issues having to do with socialization in general that need to be addressed.

These are presented in the rest of this chapter and in Chapter 2. The present chapter deals, first, with the fact that parent and child influence each other's actions, and so this back-and-forth exchange has to be unpacked in order to gain a fuller understanding of how socialization happens. Next comes a discussion of the range of values that are involved in socialization, their features, and their relation to behavior. Finally, I comment on the role of culture in socialization. Chapter 2 focuses on the most important values and the ones that have received the most research attention—those having to do with morality or concern for fairness, justice, and avoidance of harm to others, and those of concern and consideration for others. I have included this chapter because moral development has been much studied by researchers who have been concerned with either moral reasoning, moral affect, or early-appearing moral behavior. I have tried to link these three areas of inquiry—reasoning, affect, and early behavior—to some of the material covered in the rest of the book.

## ■ ESTABLISHING DIRECTION OF EFFECT OR CAUSALITY IN PARENTING RESEARCH

A great deal of research having to do with parenting and children's socioemotional development is correlational in nature. As a result, it is difficult to make assertions about whether parenting is having an impact on the child or vice versa, whether there is an exchange of influence, or whether genetic similarity provides the explanation. Children may be aggressive because they have been socialized harshly or in an aggressive manner, or parents may be harsh because their children are aggressive and harshness is the only approach that seems to work. Or a parent and child may be promoting aggressive and harsh behavior in each other. One could ask, for example, if a child is behaving badly because that child is routinely spanked for bad behavior, or whether the child, for some set of reasons, is badly behaved and drives the parent to engage in physical punishment. It would not be surprising to see that the answer involves both possibilities: The parent does not socialize the child optimally, and the resulting problematic behavior in the child leads to further deterioration in parenting practices. An additional possibility is that both parent and child are aggressive and harsh in their exchanges because they share some of the same genes. Of course, the impact of children on parents can also be positive. When children are kind and helpful, for example, this behavior may well have an effect on how their parents treat them.

Several methodological approaches can be taken to inferring direction of effect in parenting. These approaches include the collection of longitudinal data, experimental studies, and the use of findings from behavior and molecular genetic studies.

## Longitudinal Studies

In longitudinal studies, data collected at two or more time points allow the researcher to control statistically for level of behavior exhibited at an earlier time. Should there still be changes in the outcome of interest, such as a child's antisocial behavior, it can be more justifiably inferred that some feature of parenting was the cause—although it is also possible that a third, unmeasured variable linked with the parenting variable is making the causal contribution. For example, it might not be harsh parenting that is causing a child's aggression, but poverty (a variable that is linked to harsh parenting). Nevertheless, longitudinal studies are more informative than those where information is all collected at the same point in time.

## Experiments

Experiments are excellent for determining direction of effect. Their disadvantage is that it may be difficult or simply unethical to manipulate the kinds of variables that socialization theorists study. It would be a challenge, for example, to ask one randomly selected group of parents to use one form of discipline and a second group a different form, even if those forms appear to be equivalent in their desirability and acceptability. One very useful form of experimentation with respect to socialization variables, however, involves a therapeutic intervention. Parents whose children are noncompliant, for example, may seek help in modifying their children's behavior. As I describe in Chapter 4, one possible tool for promoting compliance is for parents themselves to comply with their children's reasonable requests, and this is a change in approach that can be trained. Studies described in Chapter 4 support the idea that children's compliance can be improved when parents are helped to change their approach or response to their children's reasonable wishes.

## Behavior and Molecular Genetic Studies

Because children and their parents share, on average, 50% of their genetic material, a correlation between parent behavior and child outcome could be due simply to the similarity of their genetic makeups. Findings from behavior and molecular genetic studies can be used to help make inferences about direction of effect, or even to reach a conclusion that neither member of the dyad is having a direct effect on the other. The two kinds of gene–environment associations relevant for parenting and socialization are "passive" and "evocative" gene–environment correlations.

Passive gene–environment correlations occur when parent and child share a genetic composition that is driving their own behavior; in this case, the parent is not causing the child's behavior, nor is the child causing the parent's behavior. Consider, for example, the fact that parental warmth and children's prosocial behavior are often found to be correlated (Hastings, Miller, & Troxel, 2015). The usual assumption is that parental warmth sets the conditions for children's developing sensitivity to the needs of others. However, both parental warmth and children's prosocial behavior have been shown to have a significant heritability component. Should genes for these two behaviors be present in both parents and children, then a positive relation between parental warmth and children's prosocial behavior could be attributed, in part at least, to a shared genotype rather than to parenting behavior (Knafo & Jaffee, 2013).

Another example of effects that result from shared genetic makeup comes from a study of offspring conceived with assisted reproductive technologies. In this study, investigators found that there was a correlation between smoking during pregnancy and children's development of attention-deficit/hyperactivity disorder (ADHD), but that the correlation was significantly greater when the child the mother carried was genetically related rather than unrelated (Thapar et al., 2009). These results suggest, then, that a reasonable explanation for the relation between smoking and ADHD lies in the fact that a tendency to smoke and ADHD are genetically linked, rather than smoking's being a substantial causal factor.

Other approaches demonstrating the operation of passive gene–environment correlations come from studies that find associations between a parenting variable and a child outcome in related individuals (biological parents and their children), but not in unrelated individuals (adoptive parents and their adopted children). Again, this is evidence that the direction of effect is not from parent to child, but instead that genetic similarity is driving the actions of both dyad members. Molecular genetic studies can also shed light on the direction of effect issue. For example, mothers' sensitive behavior and their children's attachment are correlated. This could reflect a causal relation between maternal sensitivity and children's feelings of security. However, variation in the oxytocin receptor gene has been associated with both maternal sensitivity and infant attachment status, thus suggesting that genetic similarity is playing a causal role in the connection between mothers' sensitivity behavior and attachment (Avinum & Knafo-Noam, 2015).

Evocative gene–environment correlations occur when children's genetically mediated behavior affects the environment or parenting that they receive. Such an effect can be established, for example, when parenting received by monozygotic twins is more similar than that received by same-sex dizygotic twins. Given that parenting is similar for monozygotic twins (who are identical in their genes), but that it differs for dizygotic twins (who share, on average, only half their genes), differences in parenting behavior have to be attributed, in part at least, to these genetic differences. Another way of studying evocative gene–environment correlations is by considering parenting in adoptive families of children with different genetic characteristics. Ge et al. (1996), for example, found that adoptive parents reacted differently to children whose biological parents had psychiatric difficulties compared to those whose biological parents did not: The former were more antisocial, and their adoptive parents were harsher. Evocative gene–environment correlations become stronger with age (Elkins, McGue, & Iacono, 1997)—a not surprising finding, given that children become more independent as they grow older and are thus in a better position to have an impact on family functioning.

## ■ VALUES AND SOCIALIZATION

"Values" are beliefs that are associated with emotion or affect and that motivate behavior. Individuals who value honesty, for example, are likely to act in an honest way because of the emotion or motivation aroused by lack of honesty. During the socialization process, parents help children learn values that manifest themselves in their children's actions. The word "help" is important, because actions and values are not simply transmitted from parent to child; they are constructed by the child, based on a whole series of events that are addressed throughout this book.

I turn now to several questions that can be asked about the learning of values:

What kinds of values do people have in general?

What values do parents think are important to teach their children?

Are some values better to teach than others with respect to their effects on children's well-being?

Are all values taught in the same way?

Are some values affected by genetic factors?

What is the relation between values and behavior?

## What Kinds of Values Do People Have?

Schwartz (1992) identified 10 basic values that human beings hold: self-direction, stimulation, hedonism, achievement, power, security, tradition, conformity, benevolence, and universalism. Their definitions are provided in Table 1.2.

The 10 values can be organized into a circular motivational continuum. Their ordering on the circle is determined by the degree of similarity or compatibility that exists between them. Values are considered to be compatible if actions that express or promote the goals of one also express or promote the goals of the other. Values are in conflict if actions that promote one do so at the expense of the other. The more compatible values are, the closer they are to each other on the circle. The more incompatible they are, the greater the distance between them on the circle. As examples, benevolence and universalism go together: The person who cares for others can also care for principles of social justice; there is no conflict here. On the other hand, the person who values achievement and power may have more difficulty espousing caring and concern for others. Thus these two values are distant from each other on the circle, because they have incompatible motivations. As people adapt to life experiences, their values change, but not in a random manner. Rather, the changes reflect the strength of a given value on the circular structure. As one value increases in importance, there

**TABLE 1.2. Definitions for Schwartz's 10 Values**

| Value | Definition |
| --- | --- |
| Self-direction | Freedom to think and act on one's own |
| Stimulation | Excitement, novelty, and change |
| Hedonism | Pleasure and sensuous gratification |
| Achievement | Success according to social standards |
| Power | Dominance through control of people and of material and social resources |
| Security | Personal and social safety |
| Tradition | Maintaining and preserving cultural, family, religious traditions |
| Conformity | Compliance with rules and avoidance of harming or upsetting others |
| Benevolence | Being reliable, trustworthy, caring toward others |
| Universalism | Commitment to equality, justice, and protection for all people and for nature |

are compensating decreases in the importance of a value on the other side of the circle.

In 2012 Schwartz and his colleagues (Schwartz et al., 2012) made some additions to the original model (see Figure 1.1). These changes consisted of more refined breakdowns of the initial values. Nevertheless, Schwartz et al. found that the ordering of the original 10 values around the circle remained more or less unchanged. Also unchanged were four higher-order values that are also shown in Figure 1.1. On opposite sides of the circle are openness to change and conservation—a positioning that reflects conflict between independence of thought and action on the one hand, and resistance to change on the other. Also on opposite sides are self-enhancement and self-transcendence—a placement that underlines the conflict between values emphasizing concern for the welfare and interests of others, and those that involve the pursuit of one's own interests and dominance.

Value hierarchies are similar across cultures (Schwartz & Bardi, 2001). Thus, in a survey of value hierarchies involving representative samples from 13 nations as well as schoolteachers in 56 nations and college students in 54 nations, benevolence consistently emerged

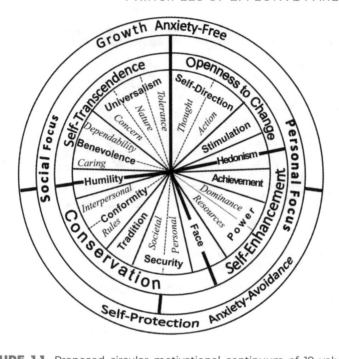

**FIGURE 1.1.** Proposed circular motivational continuum of 19 values with sources that underlie their order. From Schwartz et al. (2012). Copyright 2012 by the American Psychological Association. Reprinted by permission.

at the top of the hierarchy of values across nations, followed closely by self-direction and universalism. Security, conformity, and achievement appeared in the middle of the hierarchies, followed by hedonism. Stimulation, tradition, and power were at the bottom, with power consistently last. This does not mean that there were not differences in the degree of importance assigned to a given value in individual nations; there were such differences. There was, however, striking unanimity across cultures in the ranking of different values.

Schwartz and Bardi offered an explanation for this ranking in terms of three requirements social groups impose so that successful functioning can occur. I describe them here in order of importance. The first is the maintenance of cooperative and supportive relationships among group members in order to avoid conflict and facilitate survival; loyalty to and identification with the group and its members are essential. Thus benevolence (helpfulness, honesty, forgiveness, loyalty, responsibility) is of primary importance. Universalism is also important, but not so much as benevolence, because universalism is directed to members of the out-group (it refers to equality and protection for all) and thereby endangers in-group solidarity. (It should be noted, however, that Schwartz et al. (2012) found that universalism and benevolence had changed their relative positions.) Power is harmful to the maintenance of group solidarity and hence occupies a position at the bottom of the hierarchy. The second requirement for successful group functioning is that individuals be motivated to perform productive work, solve problems, and generate new ideas and solutions. Hence the moderate importance of achievement values. Finally, some gratification of self-oriented needs and desires is critical in order to avoid individual frustration. Thus the values of hedonism and stimulation are of some significance, although these are less likely to be promoted by social agents, because they are less relevant to group survival.

## What Values Do Parents Consider Important to Teach?

### Surveys of Parents

In a report published in 2014, 815 American parents were asked by an American polling organization (the Pew Research Center) to consider a list of 12 values and to say what they thought were the important ones to teach children. The results are summarized in Table 1.3. The number in the first column after each value is the percentage of parents who said this value was among the three most important values to teach, and the number in the second column is the percentage who said this was the most important of these three values to teach. The results indicate that being responsible, working hard, helping others, and being well mannered were most strongly endorsed as important to teach. In Schwartz's terminology, these parents had self-direction, benevolence, universalism, and conformity as primary goals for rearing their children.

### Narratives from Young Adults

In my research lab, my students and I have collected narratives from undergraduates who were asked to describe a time when they learned an important value from a parent or primary caregiver (Vinik, 2013; Vinik, Johnston, Grusec, & Farrell, 2013). The range of events our

**TABLE 1.3. Percentage of American Parents Choosing a Value as One of the Three Most Important to Teach Their Children (Column 1) and Rating a Value from That Group as Most Important (Column 2)**

| Value | Among three most important | Most important of three chosen |
|---|---|---|
| Being responsible | 94 | 54 |
| Hard work | 92 | 44 |
| Helping others | 86 | 22 |
| Being well mannered | 86 | 21 |
| Independence | 79 | 17 |
| Creativity | 72 | 10 |
| Empathy | 67 | 15 |
| Persistence | 67 | 11 |
| Tolerance | 62 | 8 |
| Obedience | 62 | 12 |
| Religious faith | 56 | 31 |
| Curiosity | 52 | 6 |

Note. Data from Pew Research Center (www.pewresearch.org/fact-tank/2014/09/18/families-may-differ-but-they-share-common-values-on-parenting).

undergraduates reported offers some additional insight into the kinds of values that parents teach. We did not ask what parents thought were important values for their children to have. Presumably, however, we were being told about values and associated actions that these undergraduates believed their parents felt to be important. The largest number of values reported by the students involved not behaving in an antisocial way (being honest, not harming others physically or psychologically)—similar to Schwartz's universalism. Next came working hard, or Schwartz's achievement. Although achievement is of only moderate importance in Schwartz's model, it was understandably of considerable importance for these first-year undergraduates. Next came looking after one's own health and safety—security, in Schwartz's terminology. Significantly different from universalism (not harming others), but no different in frequency from achievement and security, was concern/caring for others (benevolence).

## Are Some Values More Likely Than Others to Be Linked to Positive Socioemotional Outcomes?

Researchers have compared values in order to see if some are more likely than others to be associated with positive outcomes for an individual's well-being. Kasser and Ryan (1996), for example, distinguished so-called "intrinsic" from "extrinsic" values. Intrinsic values include aspirations for personal growth, meaningful relationships, social responsibility, and physical health. Extrinsic values include financial success, physical attractiveness, and social recognition. They found that intrinsic values were more likely than extrinsic values to be associated with happiness and well-being, both in a community sample of adults and in a sample of undergraduates. One explanation for this finding is provided by self-determination theory (Ryan & Deci, 2017), which posits that people need to feel that their behavior is self-determined or autonomous, rather than directed by others. Extrinsic values depend on external rewards, praise, and evaluations by others, and so those sorts of values run counter to the basic need for self-direction (Ryan & Deci, 2000). A parallel explanation is provided by Schwartz and Bardi (2001) when they argue that self-transcendent values serve successful group functioning better than self-enhancement values.

## Are All Values Taught in the Same Way?

*Moral versus Social Conventional Values*

Consider the following two problems. How do you explain to children that they shouldn't say "What the f . . k?"? And how do you explain to children that they shouldn't take a friend's toy without asking? A parent would be unlikely to give the same answer to both questions. It makes sense to say, "You shouldn't take a friend's toy without asking, because it upsets your friend, and you wouldn't like it if your friend took your toy without asking." It makes less sense to tell a child, "You shouldn't say 'What the f . . k?', because it upsets your friend, and you wouldn't like it if your friend said that to you." This comparison moves discussion into the area of domains of social knowledge (not to be confused with domains of socialization) (Turiel, 1983, 2018). Turiel and colleagues (e.g., Smetana, 2011) argue that there are different kinds of transgressions that have different origins. Among them are moral transgressions (i.e., harming others physically or psychologically) and social conventional transgressions (i.e., violation of arbitrary rules of social conduct). In the first category are actions that are inherently wrong, such as physical aggression, lying, stealing, and treating others unfairly. These are behaviors that are absolutely prohibited even if their violation produces a positive outcome for the actor. In the second category are actions that are not inherently correct but are encouraged in everyday exchanges—actions such as practicing good table manners, wearing appropriate clothing, and using polite behavior and language. The difference between the two classes of transgressions means that reasons agents of socialization offer for acceptable behavior have to be tailored to, or appropriate for, the domain in question; the same response for all misdeeds is not effective parenting. Violations of social conventions require a reference to rules and customary ways of behaving, whereas moral misdeeds require acknowledgment of the inherent immorality of an act.

## Moral versus Prosocial Values

Another distinction between different kinds of values arises when parents respond to two classes of positive social behavior. These are moral values (not harming others physically or psychologically) and prosocial values (helping or showing concern for others). Although both seem to reflect, in Schwartz's terms, universalism and benevolence, they have some distinctive properties. For example, mothers appear to react differently to antisocial behaviors (lying, stealing) and failures to be prosocial (not helping, not showing concern). They report that they are more likely to punish antisocial behaviors and to use empathic or other-oriented reasoning that focuses on the needs of others in dealing with failures to be prosocial (Grusec & Kuczynski, 1980). When asked in one study to respond to vignettes describing children's antisocial acts and children's failures to be prosocial, mothers reported that they would feel greater anger and apply more punishment in the case of antisocial acts than in the case of failures to be prosocial (Grusec, Dix, & Mills, 1982). In another study (Grusec, 1991), mothers were trained to record whenever they saw their children displaying prosocial behavior, failing to act prosocially, or failing to comply with a request for prosocial behavior, along with how the mothers and others reacted. Over the course of a month, mothers reported that children were equally likely to receive no response, acknowledgment, social approval, and praise for spontaneous prosocial behavior. When they failed to behave prosocially, mothers were more likely to respond with empathy training—that is, talking about the effects of the children's actions on others. Failures to comply with requests for prosocial behavior, in contrast, were more likely to elicit threats and nonverbal punishment—again, an indication that failure to behave in a prosocial manner is less likely to be disapproved of than moral transgressions in the form of failure to comply with a parental request. The same pattern of socialization is revealed in Vinik's (2013) finding that narratives from undergraduates describing a time when they learned a moral value (not harming others) were more likely to involve punishment and reasoning than were narratives describing a time when they learned a prosocial value.

## WHY THE DIFFERENCE?

The distinction between prosocial and moral behavior is attributable to several features of the two. Moral behavior is never wrong, given that it involves only not doing something that would harm another person. Prosocial behavior, on the other hand, is more complex. Peterson (1982) captured some of this complexity when she noted that the potential prosocial actor must learn that "I should help or give to *deserving* individuals, who are in X level of *need,* and are *dependent on me* for help, when I can *ascertain and perform* the necessary behavior and when the *cost* or *risk* to me does not exceed Y *amount* of my currently available resources" (p. 202; emphasis in original). In addition, helping others is not always correct and may be seen by recipients as a mixed blessing or even as threatening, if it makes them feel that they are inferior, failures, or dependent on others (Fisher, Nadler, & Whitcher-Alagna, 1982). Being the recipient of help also arouses feelings of obligation that are troubling, particularly if the help cannot be reciprocated. And being helpful could actually harm the recipient or have an unreasonable impact on the well-being of the donor. Trying to rescue a drowning person when one does not have the requisite skills could endanger the life of that person even more. Nor is one obligated to risk one's own life in order to save someone else's life. As a result of all these possible negative outcomes, then, it makes sense that parents would be somewhat less definite in their recommendations with respect to prosocial behavior than they are with respect to moral action.

Other features of prosocial behavior that make it more complex than moral behavior are the number of forms it takes and the number of underlying motivations that can accompany these different forms. Prosocial behavior can include helping, comforting, reassuring, and protecting, and it can be driven by a number of motives, including empathy or sympathetic concern for the distress of another, a hope of reciprocity, and/or a wish to display mastery. It may also occur because prosocial behavior has been routinized through frequent repetition so that it occurs automatically, because of a desire to act in accord with societal norms, or because concern for others is a central part of one's identity.

In view of all these complexities, then, it is not surprising that prosocial behavior and inhibition of antisocial behavior are not opposite sides of the same coin. Thus they are not correlated with each other. They also have other different correlates, with positive emotionality a predictor of prosocial behavior, and negative emotionality and lack of constraint a predictor of antisocial behavior (Krueger, Hicks, & McGue, 2001).

## Are Some Values Affected by Genetic Factors?

The question of whether some values might be affected by genetics was addressed in a study of 7-year-old Israeli twins by Uzefovsky, Döring, and Knafo-Noam (2016). The children were asked to rate the importance for them of a series of values depicted in cartoons. Benevolence, for example, was displayed in a cartoon where one child helped another who had fallen. Power was depicted by a child dressed as a king, and stimulation by a child in a parachute. Uzefovsky et al. found that (in Schwartz's terminology) values of benevolence and universalism, self-enhancement, and conformity and security were significantly affected by genetic factors, as well as by environmental experiences that were not shared by the twins. In contrast, openness to change, at least in these young children, was found to be unaffected by genetic factors and influenced by both shared and nonshared environmental factors.

## How Are Values and Behavior Related?

When and how do values manifest themselves in a child's behavior? This, of course, is the most important question for parents who are concerned with how children relate to others. Self-transcendence values have been shown to predict voluntary behavior intended to help another, whereas self-enhancement values have been shown to predict aggressive behavior (Pulfrey & Butera, 2013; Uzefovsky et al., 2016). Not only are values predictive of behavior in the immediate context, but there is also evidence that self-enhancement values are predictors of future aggression; that is, there is reason to suggest that values may be translated into action at a later point in time (Benish-Weisman, 2015). There is also evidence that behavior can play a causal role in the formation of values. For example, in a study of 10- to 12-year-olds, Vecchione, Döring, Alessandri, Marsicano, and Bardi (2016) found that over a 6-month period, values were associated with a change in behavior, and behavior was associated with a change in values. The latter outcome (behavior's predicting a change in values) was somewhat stronger than the former outcome (values' predicting a change in behavior). In essence, in order to maintain consistency between their words and deeds, these children appeared to adjust their values to match their actions. As well, engagement in particular actions may have convinced them of the merits of an underlying value.

## Internalization

Values and behavior are more likely to be linked when values have been internalized—that is, when they come to be seen by the individual as inherently correct and self-generated. Under these conditions, children (and adults) are more likely to behave well even in the absence of surveillance. Otherwise, they would have to be kept under constant scrutiny.

Georg Simmel (1902), a sociologist and philosopher, wrote the following about internalization: "The tendency of society to satisfy itself as cheaply as possible results in appeals to 'good conscience,' through which the individual pays to himself the wages for his righteousness, which otherwise would probably have to be assured to him in some way through law or custom" (p. 19). Simmel thus suggested that people reward themselves for good behavior, rather than society's having to expend valuable resources for the task. Such an arrangement is an inexpensive way for maintaining conformity with societal norms and rules. In a later discussion of internalization, Hoffman (1970a) talked about guilt as a mechanism for maintaining positive behavior, with guilt that arises from knowledge that one has harmed another being more effective in promoting positive behavior than is guilt focused on disapproval of the self.

## SELF-DETERMINATION THEORY

Considerable attention has been paid to the concept of internalization by self-determination theorists (Deci & Ryan, 1985; Ryan & Deci, 2000, 2017). They note that some behaviors, such as creative pursuits, are intrinsically motivated or inherently satisfying and enjoyable. Other behaviors, however, may not be so naturally desirable, and these are the ones that must be encouraged by agents of socialization. The motivation for these latter behaviors is located on a continuum ranging from "external" through "introjected," "identified," and "integrated." Externally regulated behavior is motivated by hope of external reward or fear of punishment. We do not take other people's belongings, or we will be punished. And we work hard at school so that our parents will be pleased. Regulation that is introjected results in actions taken to avoid guilt or anxiety or to experience feelings of pride; the behavior does not arise from a value that has been accepted as one's own and is not part of the self, and so it has not been internalized. In this case, we do not steal, not because we would be punished by our parents, but because we would punish ourselves by feeling guilty. Internalization is evident in the next two points on the continuum. Thus regulation through identification reflects a conscious valuing of a behavioral goal, such that the action is accepted as having personal importance. In this case, good behavior occurs because it is important to be honest. The final point on the continuum, integrated regulation, reflects full assimilation of a value so that it fits with the individual's other values and needs. Here the motivation for good behavior is, for example, the belief that one is a caring person who does not harm others or an honest person who always tells the truth.

According to self-determination theory, internalization occurs when three basic requirements for successful socialization are met. The first is "autonomy support." Autonomy-supportive parents provide children with choices that are developmentally appropriate, minimize the use of controls, and acknowledge the children's perspective and feelings. The second requirement is "structure," in which rationales and informational feedback are provided, and consequences are explained and consistently administered. Finally comes "relatedness," or interpersonal involvement that includes the provision of warmth and caring, devoting of time and resources to children, and taking an interest in the children's activities (Grolnick, Deci, & Ryan, 1997). These three basic requirements—autonomy support, structure, and relatedness—reappear in various forms throughout this book.

SUMMARY■ ■ ■ ■ ■ ■ ■ ■ ■ ■ ■ ■ ■ ■ ■ ■ ■ ■ ■ ■ ■ ■ ■ ■ ■ ■ ■ ■ ■ ■ ■ ■ ■ ■ ■

So what can be said about values? We know that people, on the whole, think more highly of self-transcendent values such as fairness and justice than they do of self-enhancement values such as achievement and power, both for themselves and for their children. In parallel fashion, self-transcendent values are associated with higher levels of happiness and well-being compared to self-enhancement values, presumably because the latter rely on the approval of others and so violate a basic human need for autonomy. Values are not all equivalent in other respects as well. Thus moral values, prosocial values, and social conventional values have different features and are socialized differently. And some values are more likely to be at least partially genetically mediated than are others. Finally, in order to be truly effective guides for behavior, values need to be internalized or become part of an individual's self-identity. Internalization is promoted by parental minimization of control, taking of the child's perspective, and setting of clear rules, and by a warm and caring parent–child relationship.

## ■ CULTURE AND SOCIALIZATION

Much of the research cited in this book has been carried out with children and parents from Western countries. Fortunately, research involving individuals from other parts of the world is becoming more plentiful. This expansion, of course, is vital for an understanding of socialization processes—allowing investigators, among other things, to determine what aspects of socialization are universal. Thus parental acceptance (Lansford et al., 2010), learning from parental example (Rogoff, Moore, Correa-Chavez, & Dexter, 2015), some level of personal autonomy (Helwig, 2006), and alleviation of distress in time of need (Bugental, 2000) are present in many cultures. Cultural research also allows for the identification of what is not universal and of how different parenting beliefs affect approaches to parenting. These beliefs include the nature of appropriate behavior for children, the age at which such behavior can be expected to appear, what are effective childrearing strategies, and the meaning of different parenting interventions. I consider each of these in turn.

Parents in different cultural contexts can have different goals, depending on the behaviors they believe their children need to display in order to get along well with others in their society or group.

One frequently cited example is the extent to which autonomy from the group is stressed as opposed to interdependence, with these two features often characterized as an "individualist" versus "collectivist" orientation. The former emphasizes children's self-esteem and confidence, whereas the latter emphasizes being part of the group and having respect for elders (Markus & Kitayama, 1991). These different orientations lead to different parenting practices and different child outcomes. For example, although agents of socialization emphasize prosocial behavior regardless of culture (Schwartz & Bardi, 2001), the way in which it is encouraged can vary. Thus American undergraduates value spontaneous prosocial behavior, whereas Hindu Indian undergraduates place greater emphasis on the importance of responding to a request or on reciprocity (Miller & Bersoff, 1994). Similarly, when responding to moral dilemmas, Hindu Indians are more likely to give priority to interpersonal responsibilities, whereas Americans are more likely to respond with considerations for justice (Miller & Bersoff, 1992).

Cultures also differ in their expectations with respect to developmental timetables. Japanese mothers, for example, expect their children to be able to control their emotions, be polite, and comply with adult requests at younger ages than do American mothers, whereas American mothers expect their children to be assertive and to master social skills at younger ages than do Japanese mothers (Hess, Kashiwagi, Azume, Price, & Dickson, 1980). Yet another distinction among cultural groups has to do with beliefs about effective childrearing practices. These include the way in which parental authority should be implemented, the amount of autonomy that should be granted, and whether children should be played with (Bornstein, 2007; Chao, 1994; Harkness & Super, 1996). Keller et al. (2006), for example, have shown how mother–child interactions are differently structured in different groups, with Western babies having more face-to-face interactions (a distal interaction style), and rural African children being more likely to have greater body contact (a proximal interaction style). The two styles, then, reflect different views of the self: as either autonomous and separate, or interdependent and compliant.

A final example of cultural effects has to do with the meaning assigned to a particular intervention. Chao (1994, 2001), for example, has pointed out that authoritarian parenting has a different meaning in Asian cultures than it does in Western ones. In Western cultures, it signifies lack of autonomy support and of caring responsiveness. In Asian cultures, it means "training"; strict parental control is seen as a manifestation of parental involvement, concern for the child's future, and caring and love. As a result, the consequences of authoritarian parenting are different and less negative in Asian than in Western contexts.

Cultural comparisons are important. Nevertheless, it is also essential to remember that there is substantial variability in socialization practices within each culture, and that this may even surpass variability between cultures (Carlo, Roesch, Knight, & Koller, 2001). Immigration increases the heterogeneity of parenting in Western countries, and globalization introduces Western ideas to other parts of the world. Moreover, the attitudes and beliefs of individuals who decide to immigrate may well be different from those who do not. Thus a Chinese Canadian or a Lebanese American may well differ not only from a Canadian or American of Western European descent, but from Chinese or Lebanese individuals still living in their home country.

## ■ MOVING ON

Most of the remainder of this book is devoted to how the internalization of values is best achieved, with the argument that this internalization is accomplished in different ways in different domains of social functioning. The focus is on agents of socialization and, in particular, on what the research evidence reveals about their role in socialization. Before moving into this discussion, however, I devote the next chapter to a discussion of two singularly important values—moral and prosocial (or universalism and benevolence). I do this because so much has been written about the development of these forms of positive social behavior, as well as about the reasoning and affect associated with them, that it is important to see how those writings fit with or contribute to an understanding of domains of socialization.

# CHAPTER 2

# Moral Values, Reasoning, Affect, and Action

Although parents teach children a wide range of values, socialization theorists have focused on two classes of values in particular: moral and prosocial. As a result, considerable research has been devoted to how not harming others—and, less frequently, how showing concern for others—can be encouraged in young children. This particular interest in moral and prosocial development has not been confined to researchers who study parenting and socialization processes, however. In this chapter, I briefly survey some other approaches to the learning of values, primarily focused on moral development, and link them to the concerns of socialization researchers. The three lines of investigation include studies of moral development and reasoning; moral development and its relation to emotion; and intuitive, or very early, morality. I discuss these, in part at least, because there is often confusion when people talk about moral development as to what aspect they have in mind. Also important, of course, is how these approaches intersect with each other and what one can contribute to an understanding of the others, as well as to socialization theory.

## ■ MORAL DEVELOPMENT AND REASONING

Cognitive developmental theorists have focused on reasoning about moral issues and have examined how that reasoning moves from a concern with avoidance of punishment to a sophisticated level of reasoning that revolves around abstract principles of justice. Their approach differs from that of socialization theorists in what they see as the antecedents of moral development, the role of parents in moral development, and the relation between moral reasoning and moral behavior. The major figures associated with this approach are Jean Piaget, Lawrence Kohlberg, and Elliot Turiel.

## Jean Piaget

In *The Moral Judgment of the Child,* Piaget (1932) described children's construction of morality both in their play and in their responses to stories about children misbehaving. In the stage of what Piaget called "heteronomous" morality, whether or not an act is deemed unacceptable depends on the amount of damage done: For instance, a boy who breaks 15 cups accidentally is worse than one who breaks a single cup while stealing jam. In the next stage, that of "autonomous" morality, intention becomes a factor, and now the boy who breaks one cup while stealing is considered to be behaving more unacceptably than the one who accidentally breaks many cups. Development also occurs with respect to whether or not rules can be changed. For young children, rules are unalterable; for older ones, they can be modified if there is group support. In Piaget's analysis, movement from a less to a more mature stage of development is enabled by decreases in egocentrism and increases in the ability to take the perspective of others. An additional factor contributing to the development of more mature reasoning is that of increasing opportunities for peer interaction, because, in Piaget's view, the authoritarian relationship between parent and child provides fewer opportunities for consideration of alternative views than do the more egalitarian relationships afforded by peers. Finally, Piaget was not interested in behavior, and so he had little to say about any links between the level of a child's moral reasoning and that child's actions.

## Lawrence Kohlberg

Kohlberg's (1976) stages of moral development are well known by anyone interested in moral development. As Piaget did, Kohlberg emphasized reasoning and not behavior, and he made no attempt to link reasoning and action. As well, in agreement with Piaget, Kohlberg saw the development of more and more sophisticated reasoning as dependent on the child's increasing abilities to think logically and to take the perspective of others, rather than on parental teaching.

In his research, Kohlberg collected responses to a series of stories involving moral dilemmas. In one often-cited story, Heinz's wife is dying and needs expensive medication. Heinz borrows half the necessary money and asks the druggist if he may pay the rest of the money later. The druggist refuses, and so Heinz steals the drug. The important question for Kohlberg was not whether stealing the drug is good or bad, or what Heinz should do, but *why* stealing the drug is good or bad.

Kohlberg found that moral reasoning could be categorized into three levels with two stages at each level. These six stages involve increasingly sophisticated reasons for why actions are appropriate or inappropriate. Moral reasoning begins at the "preconventional" level with, in the first stage, discussions of punishment avoidance: People should behave in a way that does not get them into trouble with others. Thus Heinz is right to steal the drug because it is not worth that much, or he should not steal the drug because stealing is a crime and therefore punishable. The second stage, still at the preconventional level, involves reciprocity: People should behave well so others will behave well toward them in turn. Reasoning moves next to the level of "conventional" morality. Here appropriate behavior, at the third stage, is that which pleases others and gains their approval: Heinz is right to steal the drug because he loves his wife, or he is wrong to steal it because he has tried everything he can possibly do to save her life. The fourth stage involves the importance of maintaining respect for authority and the social order. Finally, at the level of "postconventional" morality, good behavior is that which has been decided on by society (fifth stage), or behavior is determined on the basis of ethical principles chosen by the self and based on justice and respect for human dignity (sixth stage). In this last stage, Heinz is right to steal because the higher principle is saving human lives; or he is wrong to steal because one should not act on the basis of emotion or the law, but on the basis of what is the most just action, and theft of the drug may not have been most just. In sum, then, reasons or motivations for good behavior move from a concern with external consequences to a focus on self-chosen or internalized principles. This movement seems quite parallel to movement along the motivational continuum described by self-determination theorists (and briefly summarized in Chapter 1), which begins with external motivation and ends with internalized principles.

Kohlberg (1976) found that the first two stages of reasoning were typical of children up to about the age of 9 years, some adolescents, and adult criminal offenders. The next two stages were typical of most adults, and the last two stages of a few adults. Kohlberg also found that these stages occurred in an invariant order and that none was skipped (Colby, Kohlberg, Gibbs, & Lieberman, 1983). The conclusion that the order of stages does not vary receives further support from findings that the training of moral thinking is most successful when arguments are presented at one stage above the current stage at which a student is functioning (Turner & Berkowitz, 2005). Finally, Kohlberg maintained that basic moral judgment is universal—a conclusion that is generally seen as correct, at least in principle (Gibbs, Basinger, Grime, & Snarey, 2007). Thus, in a large number of cultural contexts, there is evidence for basic moral judgment development and related social perspective taking, even if specific manifestations of this development are influenced by differing beliefs and practices.

### Reasoning about Prosocial Behavior

Kohlberg's theory deals with the reasons people have for refraining from antisocial acts such as stealing, lying, or harming others. Eisenberg (e.g., Eisenberg, Lennon, & Roth, 1983) used Kohlberg's approach as a model for understanding reasoning about prosocial actions such as concern for others. She and her colleagues identified five levels of prosocial reasoning that map to an extent on Kohlberg's levels of moral reasoning. Notably missing from Eisenberg's catalogue of levels is reference to external prohibitions—an omission that fits well, of course, with my observation in Chapter 1 that failure to behave prosocially is rarely punished. Eisenberg's stages of prosocial reasoning begin with a hedonistic concern for one's own needs: "I'd help him because I like him," or "I'd help him because he could help me another time." Next is an orientation to the needs of others: The reason for assistance is expressed simply in terms of someone's needing help. The third stage reveals a stereotyped approval-focused orientation, in which one helps to impress others or to be liked. Next comes the expression of genuine empathy, as children take the perspective of others and assist them because they share their distress. The final stage reflects an internalized orientation, in which prosocial behavior reflects internalized values and responsibilities, and reasons involve reference to one's own set of principles.

## Elliot Turiel

Kohlberg's theory has been challenged by Turiel and his colleagues (e.g., Turiel, 1983; Smetana, 1997), who point out that even very young children have a sense of morality that develops well before middle childhood, and that they can reason in a way that is genuinely moral. In a "domains-of-social-knowledge" approach (introduced in Chapter 1), these investigators describe three categories of values: moral values related to physical or psychological harm to others, such as lying, stealing, or hurting other people's feelings; social conventional values, such as table manners, proper forms of address, or dressing appropriately, which comprise rules or conventions for facilitating smooth social interactions; and "prudential" values, or values associated with personal safety and well-being. These values, unlike stages of moral reasoning, are not developmentally ordered as a function of increasing cognitive sophistication. Rather, they are constructed by children as they interact with their environment. For example, young children are quite often victims as well as perpetrators of physical or psychological harm, and so they quickly learn the universally negative impact of these events. Social conventions take longer to learn or construct, because they are less likely to attract disapproval from peers, usually requiring input from adults (Smetana, 1997). Even preschoolers, however, can distinguish between moral and social conventional transgressions. They judge moral dictates to be unalterable and moral transgressions to be wrong, even in the absence of formally stated rules and independent of what authority figures might dictate. Social conventional rules such as talking during naptime or not standing in line, on the other hand, are judged to be contingent on the presence of rules and subject to the wishes of authority figures (Smetana, 1981). Parenting also plays a role in the learning of these distinctions. Dahl and Campos (2013), for example, found that mothers' responses to questions about how they would deal with the transgressions of their toddlers differed systematically as a function of the domain of child misbehavior: Physical restraint and reasoning involving harm to others were more frequent in the moral domain, and commands were more frequent in the prudential domain. Dahl, Sherlock, Campos, and Theunissen (2014) also observed that mothers altered their tone of voice depending on the nature of their toddler's misbehavior. They were more likely to use intense and angry vocalizations in response to moral transgressions, fearful or comforting vocalizations in response to prudential transgressions, and comforting vocalizations in response to pragmatic (for example, spilling a drink). These early-differentiated responses by parents precede the age at which children have been shown to make explicit distinctions among domains of social knowledge, and thus may be a central part of the mechanism by which the distinctions are developed.

Again, in the domains-of-social-knowledge approach, the emphasis is on reasoning and cognition, although less on the role of perspective taking and logical thinking. Parents are not seen to play a central role in the development of moral character, although they may have some input. Nor is there any suggestion that moral thinking will automatically lead to moral behavior, given the complexity of the considerations often involved in choice of action. Another feature of the approach is that moral knowledge is seen to be constructed by children themselves, rather than being transmitted unaltered from adults to children. The latter view stems from psychoanalytic notions of introjection or internalization and is discussed in Chapter 5.

## ▰ MORAL EMOTIONS AND MORAL ACTION

### Moral Emotions

Piaget, Kohlberg, and Turiel were all interested in moral thinking or reasoning, rather than moral emotion and action. Morality, however, has a large affective or emotional component that plays a central role in its development; knowing why something is morally wrong and feeling that something is morally wrong are not the same thing (Baird, 2008). Moral emotions are complex. They include empathy, sympathy, guilt, and shame. The ways in which they relate to moral reasoning and moral action, and the ways these relations change over the course of development, have been the objects of investigation by yet another group of researchers who study moral development.

### *Empathy and Sympathy*

"Empathy" involves the sharing of another person's emotional experience. As an example, when individuals see someone crying, they may be moved to tears as well. Empathy occurs because watching someone else experiencing an emotion or sensation activates some of the same neural substrates that are operative when the self experiences that same emotion or sensation (Decety, 2011). "Sympathy," in contrast to empathy, emerges only after children are able to distinguish between themselves and others; it refers to feelings of concern for the distress or bad fortune of others, but not an actual sharing of their emotion (Eisenberg, Fabes, & Spinrad, 2006). The intensity and frequency of sympathy increase as middle childhood is reached (Eisenberg, Spinrad, & Knafo-Noam, 2015). Some of this increase is no doubt a reflection of parenting that involves the use of reasoning focused on the feelings and needs of others, as well as the modeling of prosocial behavior. More sophisticated perspective-taking skills also contribute to the increase in sympathy as contact with peers increases.

### Guilt

"Guilt" has been defined as a feeling of regret over wrongdoing, leading to a desire to punish the self or to make recompense (Ferguson & Stegge, 1998). Recall that Hoffman (1970a) made a distinction between two forms of guilt. The first is "humanistic" guilt and involves concern for the impact of one's behavior on the welfare of others, as well as a consideration of extenuating circumstances with respect to that behavior. The second, "conventional" guilt, includes rigid adherence to institutional norms, regardless of consequences. He found that children who exhibited humanistic guilt, compared to those who exhibited conventional guilt, were more tolerant of antisocial impulses and more likely to experience guilt as a direct result of awareness of the effect of their behavior on others. Conventional children, on the other hand, were more apt to deny or repress antisocial impulses and more likely to experience guilt as resulting from their own impulse expression rather than from the harm done to others. It follows, then, that humanistic guilt would be more likely to promote internalization of values, because knowledge of having harmed others can never be escaped. Conventional guilt, in contrast, is under the control of the self and can be ignored.

### Shame

In contrast to guilt, "shame" is a negative feeling that focuses on devaluing aspects of the entire self and is often associated with the wish to change certain aspects or features of one's self (Eisenberg, 2000). When individuals experience shame, they feel bad about themselves, as opposed to feeling bad about a specific misdeed they may have committed. Shame can also be felt when someone with whom there is close identification, such as a family member, friend, or close associate, behaves in an unacceptable way. This is because their behavior is a reflection of deficiencies in one's own self. Children who behave badly, for example, can bring shame on their family members, who presumably were unable to teach them appropriate ways of getting along with others (Lickel, Schmader, Curtis, Scarnier, & Ames, 2005).

## Linking Emotion Attributions and Action

An important series of studies for understanding the relation between emotion and action involve what is known as the "happy-victimizer" effect (Barden, Zelko, Duncan, & Masters, 1980; Arsenio, 1988). In a happy-victimizer story, children are told about other children who have been wronged by, for example, having had something they value stolen from them. Five-year-olds, although they know that the thief's action was wrong, nevertheless say that the thief is happy. Older children are more likely to attribute negative emotions to the thief, because their emotion and moral reasoning now coincide. Of particular interest is the fact that older children who continue to suggest that perpetrators of immoral behavior feel some happiness are also more likely to be aggressive than those who have made the more appropriate connection between affect and reasoning (Arsenio, 2014). In this case, then, the appropriate joining of affect and action has not taken place.

The relation between emotion attributions and behavior was investigated in a survey of the literature by Malti and Krettanauer (2013). Their meta-analysis involved 42 studies and more than 8,000 participants between the ages of 4 and 10 years; it revealed significant associations between moral emotion attributions such as guilt and happiness, and both prosocial and antisocial behavior. Anticipation of feeling a particular emotion, then, is clearly a determinant of subsequent action. Interestingly, Malti and Krettanauer found that results were somewhat stronger for antisocial behavior than for prosocial behavior—a finding in accordance with the conclusion that failure to engage in prosocial behavior is less likely to be disciplined, thereby leading to a negative emotion, than is the commission of antisocial acts.

## Affect, Reasoning, and Brain Activation

Neuroscientists have weighed in on the issue of how and when emotion and cognition are related. In one study, for example, Decety, Michalska, and Kinzler (2011) asked individuals between the ages of 4 and 37 years to look at and make judgments about scenarios depicting intentional and accidental harm. They found that moral evaluation involves a complex integration of emotion and cognition that changes with age. Thus brain structures involved in emotion (the amygdala and insula) decrease in activation in response to moral issues with age, and structures involved with decision making and evaluation (the ventromedial prefrontal cortex) increase in activation in response to moral content with age. Structures involved with decision making and evaluation also become more coupled with structures associated with emotion. Decety et al. concluded that negative emotion alerts individuals to a moral challenge by making them uncomfortable, and that their discomfort then becomes a precursor of moral judgment and decision making.

## ■ INTUITIVE MORALITY

Yet a third group of researchers interested in moral development have suggested that the ability of humans to make moral judgments is rooted in intuition—that is, in automatic responses to morally relevant actions. These automatic responses have an emotional component, and they do not involve reasoning (see reviews by Wynn & Bloom, 2014; Vaish & Tomasello, 2014; Van de Vondervoort & Hamlin, 2016). Thus studies of infants and very young children indicate that even preverbal children have some understanding of moral issues, and that this understanding is independent of conscious reasoning. What is the source of these intuitions? One possibility is that humans have evolved to be sensitive to the moral actions of others, because this sensitivity benefits their survival and reproductive success. Thus it becomes important to assess the likelihood that other individuals may cooperate, and to avoid or have negative feelings toward those who are uncooperative or who behave unfairly or hurtfully.

In one study (Hamlin & Wynn, 2011), infants saw a puppet trying unsuccessfully to climb a hill, retrieve a ball, or open a box. Then they saw another puppet who was either helpful (e.g., pushed the first puppet up the hill) or hurtful (e.g., pushed the first puppet down the hill).

By the age of 3 months, infants preferred a helpful puppet, as assessed by the amount of time they looked at it; when only slightly older, they reached for the puppet who helped more than the puppet who hindered. Other research has shown that there is a moral element to these preferences, with infants by about the age of 8 months preferring a puppet who intended to be helpful even if that help was not successful (Behne, Carpenter, & Tomasello, 2005). As well, infants prefer puppets who help a puppet who previously has behaved prosocially, as well as preferring puppets who hinder a puppet who previously has behaved in a hurtful way. In other words, infants endorse the reward of moral individuals and the punishment of wrongdoers (Hamlin, 2014).

In addition to these sorts of preferences, very young children exhibit an impressive array of positive social actions (Vaish & Tomasello, 2014). They help others by, for example, picking up an object an adult has accidentally dropped, or opening a cabinet door for an adult whose arms are full, or pointing out an object for which the adult is searching. As well, they can provide comfort and reassurance when someone is in distress. As early as 8 months of age, infants show empathy by facial, vocal, and gestural manifestations of concern for others experiencing distress. Moreover, prosocial behavior in the form of attempts at comfort that appear in the second year are predicted by differences in empathy assessed in the first year (Roth-Hanania, Davidov, & Zahn-Waxler, 2011). Very young children also are more inclined to help others who have helped them (Dunfield & Kuhlmeier, 2010), indicating early sensitivity to reciprocity. Less clear is the extent to which toddlers understand the notions of sharing and of fair or equal distribution of resources—aspects of moral behavior not strongly related to empathic capacities.

Vaish and Tomasello (2014) argue that early moral actions have their base in the human need for collaboration and interdependence. They suggest, however, that this early understanding of morality is one based on personal relationships and social emotions, rather than on more general principles or norms concerning appropriate or moral behavior that are independent of specific situations and people. The latter begin to develop during the preschool years. In a summary of these developmental changes, Vaish and Tomasello note that preschoolers begin to notice at about the age of 3 years when buttons are missing, trash is on the floor, or pages in a book are torn. They apply words such as "broken," "dirty," and "bad" to situations where something is wrong, as well as react negatively and emotionally to these situations (Kagan, 1982). Importantly, their reactions occur not just when something bad has happened to themselves, but when something bad or hurtful happens to someone or something else. Three-year-olds protest when one puppet threatens to steal or throw away another puppet's possessions, whereas 2-year-olds do not. Three-year-olds return stolen objects to their rightful owners. They also protest when there is violation of a social conventional norm: For instance, games must be played according to the rules. In accord with the distinction between forms of social knowledge, 3-year-olds disapprove universally when moral norms are violated, but protest more strongly when social conventional norms are violated by members of their own group than by members of another group (Schmidt, Rakoczy, & Tomasello, 2011). All these findings, then, point to the early development of generalized norms for moral action that are universally applied to all members of one's social group, and that form a substantial base for the task of socialization.

As a result of the findings just described, a number of theorists have argued that morality is part of human nature, and that these early moral and prosocial behaviors cannot be results of socialization (Brownell & Early Social Development Research Lab, 2016). Brownell argues, however, that socialization of moral behaviors occurs continuously by means of social interaction that begins at birth. Infants are equipped with an eagerness to take part in social and emotional exchanges, and these bidirectional exchanges are what form the basis of positive motives and action. The fact that human infants have a stable supine posture frees their hands and allows them to engage in face-to-face communication and a shared focus on objects. All this encourages social and emotional development, including respect and concern for others and shared experiences. Added to this early-appearing feature of caregiver–child interaction is the fact that parents begin to socialize positive social behavior very early in life.

## SUMMARY ■ ■ ■ ■ ■ ■ ■ ■ ■ ■ ■ ■ ■ ■ ■ ■ ■ ■ ■ ■ ■ ■ ■ ■ ■ ■ ■ ■ ■ ■ ■ ■ ■ ■

Moral development has a long history of investigation by developmental psychologists who were less interested in the topic of this book—how parents socialize children to behave in accord with societal norms—than in how children and adults think about moral issues. Kohlberg was not so much interested in the exact nature of behavioral choices as he was in the increasing sophistication of reasons given for

choices. He found that early reasoning involves the avoidance of punishment and the hope of having actions reciprocated. Later reasoning
reflects abstract principles of justice and fairness, or what is referred
to as "internalization." Kohlberg's reasons resemble the reasons for
positive social behavior outlined by self-determination theorists (see
Chapter 1), beginning with external rationales and moving on to more
abstract principles or motivations for action. Both Piaget and Kohlberg argued that increasing cognitive sophistication, such as the ability
to take the perspective of others, underlies the development of moral
reasoning. Neither of them saw much room for parenting or socialization in the course of that development. Indeed, Piaget suggested that
parents' authority relationship with their children impedes children's
ability to take the perspective of others. Self-determination theorists,
on the other hand, emphasize parental autonomy support, structure,
and relatedness as aspects of parenting behavior that affect the motivation or reason for children's socially desirable actions.

Turiel's emphasis was also on increasing cognitive sophistication and the way in which children construct values from their daily
experiences. Importantly, his distinction between classes of values has
major implications for approaches to socialization: What is an effective
approach depends on the kind of value under consideration. Moral values, because of their inherent correctness, are very easily learned from
an early age when children experience personally the consequences
of immoral acts. The move from recognizing that certain actions are
immoral to behaving in accord with that recognition, of course, is the
challenge. And it is this challenge that is faced by socialization theorists.

A necessary tool in the development of positive social behavior is
affect or emotion. Empathy and sympathy for the plight of another are
powerful motivators of moral and prosocial behavior. Guilt (in its various forms) and shame are also drivers of action, pushing the individual
to translate a value into behavior. How these emotions become motivators of positive social behavior is, again, the challenge for socialization
researchers.

Recent intriguing findings with respect to early examples of
moral and prosocial behavior—responding in a caring and concerned
way to someone else's distress, helping, preferring others who behave
morally—underline the innate desire of humans to reach out to each
other in a positive and caring way. Thus this intuitive morality provides
a base on which socialization processes can build.

## ■ MOVING ON

In this chapter, I have dealt with the values of not harming others and, to a lesser extent, of showing concern for and helping others. I have chosen these particular values because they are rated high in importance (see Chapter 1); because they are the values most studied by developmentalists; and because it is useful to see how researchers have approached their investigation, and how the results of their research might fit in with an understanding of the socialization process. In the remainder of this book, I discuss a wider range of values and what is known about how those values are learned and translated into action. The discussion is organized into the five domains in which socialization takes place. The first two, protection and reciprocity, focus on the relationship between parent and child and on how that facilitates value learning; the next three focus on ways in which specific messages about values are relayed. Good relationships form a base for, and facilitate the successful learning of, messages.

# CHAPTER 3

# The Protection Domain

## *Responsiveness to Distress and Security*

The protection domain involves the formation of one kind of parent–child relationship, with the quality of this relationship ultimately affecting the child's learning of values. The theoretical base for this domain consists of attachment theory and the singularly important aspect of parent–child relationship quality—how caregivers respond to their child's distress and need for safety. In this domain, parents assume the roles of defenders from danger, providers of comfort, and secure bases from which the world can be explored. When parents provide adequate protection, their children trust that those parents have their best interests at heart. Parents operating in the protection domain must also teach children how to take over the role of protectors for themselves. In this way, then, children learn how to keep safe on their own, as well as how to cope with disturbing events.

Early work by attachment theorists included a focus on children's compliance. Taking an evolutionary perspective, for example, Stayton, Hogan, and Ainsworth (1971) argued that as infants and young children explore the world, they need to comply with parental demands that keep them safe in the case of danger. Accordingly, the human species has evolved so that children have a predisposition to comply with parental directives and warning signals, and to seek proximity to a safe and secure base. For many animals, the safe base or place of retreat is a nest or burrow. For the human species, it is the caregiver.

Research on the influence of early parenting experiences on the development of children's empathy, sympathy, and concern for others is also relevant for understanding socialization in the protection domain. Thus, in the course of teaching children to cope with distress on their own, caregivers facilitate the growth of empathy ("emotional contagion," or an emotional capacity that involves the sharing of another's emotional experience), sympathy (a feeling of concern for the other that does not involve experiencing the same or similar emotions as the other), and prosocial behavior.

## ■ ORIGINS OF ATTACHMENT THEORY

Two people, John Bowlby and Mary Ainsworth, have been the central players in attachment theory's development. I begin with an overview of some of their important contributions.

### John Bowlby

Attachment theory grew out of an evolutionary perspective, but also a psychoanalytic one, specifically, object relations theory. Object relations theory was proposed in the early 1900s when some psychoanalytically oriented thinkers (e.g., Klein, 1952) argued that the ways people relate to others and to situations in their adult lives are shaped by family experiences during infancy. Their behavior, however, is not motivated by sexual and aggressive drives, as Freud suggested. Nor is it the result of caregivers' becoming secondarily reinforcing because they have been paired with the satisfaction of primary drives such as hunger and thirst, as suggested by social learning theorists. Rather, it is driven primarily by the need for contact with others and for the formation of relationships with them. Bowlby was influenced by these ideas (Klein was his supervisor at the British Psychoanalytic Institute). Additionally, he was aware of the work of Lorenz (1935/1970) on "imprinting"—the instinctive bonding by geese and other prosocial birds, within the first hours of hatching, with the first moving object that they see. The phenomenon of imprinting clearly indicated that social bond formation need not be tied to feeding—another argument against the social learning position. Later, as well, Bowlby was influenced by Harlow's work with rhesus monkeys (Harlow, 1958; Harlow & Zimmermann, 1958; Seay & Harlow, 1965). This work included striking demonstrations of monkeys preferring to cling to cloth-covered rather than wire-covered surrogate mothers, even when the wire mothers were sources of food and the cloth-covered ones were not. Harlow also studied the devastating effects of maternal separation in rhesus monkeys, and this interest aligned with Bowlby's interest in human mother–child separation.

Bowlby's first empirical study, based on his case notes from the London Child Guidance Clinic, was published in 1944. Many of the patients he saw at the clinic had difficulties with emotional expression and were prone to antisocial behavior. By examining a large number of these cases, he was able to link their symptoms to histories of maternal deprivation and separation. In 1948, Bowlby hired James Robertson to join him in an observational study of hospitalized and institutionalized children who were separated from their parents. Robertson was a conscientious objector during World War II and had worked as a boilerman in Anna Freud's Hampstead residential nursery for children who were homeless. Here he was trained by Freud to record his observations of the children's behavior, which then became the basis for weekly group discussions (Bretherton, 1992). The training made Robertson a perfect candidate for the work with Bowlby. Robertson (1953) subsequently made a film, *A Two-Year-Old Goes to Hospital*, which followed a young girl as she was hospitalized for a minor operation (see also Bowlby & Robertson, 1953). The film vividly depicted her unhappiness at separation from her mother—unhappiness not noticed by the busy hospital staff, in part because of her quiet demeanor. It followed her as she moved from protest to anger and then despair. The film led to widespread changes in hospital procedures, because it clearly demonstrated the consequences of separation from an attachment figure, particularly under stressful conditions.

Robertson made a number of other films dealing with issues of mother–child separation. Here is a synopsis of *John, 17 Months*, the story of a young child who spent 9 days in a residential nursery (*www. robertsonfilms.info/john.htm*):

John is a loved child who has never been out of his mother's care. At 17 months he is admitted to a group of toddlers in a residential nursery while his mother is in hospital to have a second child. The nurses are young and friendly, but the system of group care does not allow any one of them to substitute for the absent mother. John tries hard to make a relationship to get the comfort he needs, but he is defeated and becomes increasingly distressed.

The cheerful young nurses are habituated to sporadic crying, and as they are not assigned to the care of individual children the severity of John's distress is not recognised until a late stage; even then, the work-system prevents the child's need of substitute mothering from being met. When on the ninth day John's mother comes to take him home, he will not accept her and struggles to get out of her arms. He looks at his mother in a way she has never seen before.

## Bowlby and Mothers

In the discussion that follows, reference is predominantly to mothers. Clearly, both Bowlby and Ainsworth considered the mother–child attachment as primary and basic, and that with the father or other caregivers as less central to the child's socioemotional development. Of course, the marked changes that have occurred in the last several decades with respect to fathers' role in childrearing indicate that this focus on mothers is becoming less appropriate. Indeed, the importance of father–child relationships is increasingly recognized in custody arrangements after divorce: Joint custody of children has become a much more frequent alternative to custody by one parent, usually the mother. Children also develop attachment relationships with teachers and other caregiving relatives, and research findings from studies of Israeli children raised on a kibbutz indicate that the *metapelet*—the communal caregiver—may be a greater source of attachment-related behavior than the biological parent (Oppenheim, Sagi, & Lamb, 1988).

## Bowlby's Theory of Attachment

According to Bowlby's (1969) analysis of attachment, humans, among other species, have evolved to favor maintenance of a close physical relationship between mother and child. As a result, the young can be protected from dangerous and life-threatening situations, and therefore are more likely to survive. In this way, reproductive success is achieved, because parents who protect their children so they can live to reproduce have ensured that their own genes will remain in the gene pool. Attachment is the mechanism whereby proximity leads to survival.

Bowlby identified two features of the child's attachment system. The first is exploration. Infants and toddlers need to explore their world, and this exploration is facilitated if they have a secure base to which they know they can return if they feel anxious or uncomfortable. The second is fear, which is activated when a child experiences a situation such as illness, distress, or a clue to danger (e.g., darkness, a loud noise, being alone, or a sudden movement in the immediate environment). When fear is experienced, the attachment system is aroused, and the child moves back toward the attachment or protective figure. According to Bowlby (1969), "In every description of primate infants in the wild, it is reported that at the least alarm an infant away from its mother will rush to her and that one already near her will cling more tightly. That attachment behavior is exhibited without fail on such occasions is of utmost importance for our understanding of both cause and function" (p. 196).

How effectively an attachment figure can serve in the role of protector depends on the quality of social interaction between parent and child, especially the attachment figure's sensitivity and responsiveness to the infant's signals. The importance of such sensitivity and responsiveness is recognized in the following analogy attributed to Bowlby by Ainsworth, Blehar, Waters, and Wall (1978):

> The safety of an army in the field depends both on its defense against attack and on maintaining a line of communications with its base. Should the field commander judge that retreat is the best tactic, it is essential the base be available to him, that he not be cut off from it, and that the commander in charge of the base be trusted to maintain the base and the support implicit in it. By analogy, the young child may be afraid of the threat implicit in the clues to danger he perceives in a situation, but he may also be afraid if he doubts the accessibility of his "base"—his attachment figure. (p. 20)

Bowlby (1973) went on to note that if the attachment figure acknowledges the child's need for comfort and protection, and respects the child's need for independent exploration of the environment, the outcome is a positive one: The child develops an "internal working model" of the self as valued and self-reliant. On the other hand, for a child whose parent has frequently rejected the need for exploration or for comfort, the result is an internal working model of the self as incompetent or as unworthy. These working models then influence the way in which that child subsequently interacts with the parent. Thus the type of working model that is constructed is of great importance for subsequent development.

In addition to the attachment system, Bowlby talked about a "sociable" system, which, he argued, is quite distinct from the attachment system. The sociable system focuses on many people, not just one person in particular, and reflects a desire to be near people in general, as opposed to the desire to be near one person—the attachment object. In fact, the sociable system is not activated when the attachment system has been aroused. Thus children who are distressed or anxious are not terribly interested in enjoying the company of others.

Yet another system involves the caregiver. The primary event in this system is retrieval of the child by the caregiver; it also includes the caregiver's reaching for, grasping, restraining, following, soothing, and rocking the child (George & Solomon, 1996). Babies have evolved to keep their caregivers close. They are physically appealing with large heads and small noses, and these features, along with their smiles and cries, keep their parents in close attendance. In this way, nature has made it more certain that a child's attachment figure is nearby and available for protection. Indeed, when a parent is not in the caregiving mode, the baby is less likely to explore. That is why when a mother's attention is diverted from her baby (e.g., when she is given a magazine to read), her baby's exploring decreases (Sorce & Emde, 1981).

Other systems beyond the caregiving one can be activated in the parent. For example, parents also act as playmates or as teachers (or, to use the terminology of this book, operate in the reciprocity or guided learning domains). Moreover, parents can be more comfortable or perform better in some of these systems than in others. A mother may be a good playmate, for example, or an excellent teacher, but a poor source of comfort when the attachment system is activated.

## SUMMARY ■ ■ ■ ■ ■ ■ ■ ■ ■ ■ ■ ■ ■ ■ ■ ■ ■ ■ ■ ■ ■ ■ ■ ■ ■ ■ ■ ■ ■ ■ ■ ■ ■ ■ ■ ■

The attachment system involves two parts: the child's desire to explore and learn, and the child's fear in response to a dangerous situation. When fear is aroused, the attachment system is activated, and the child turns to the attachment object for comfort and protection. Caregivers who encourage exploration and who provide appropriate comfort when necessary have children who develop a model of the self as valued and self-reliant. In addition to the attachment system, and different from it, is the sociable system, which involves a desire to be near others but not as sources of comfort. Mothers also have their own systems.

One is caregiving, which keeps them close to their children in order to protect them. They also play with their children and act as teachers. Finally, mothers vary in how well they perform when these different systems are activated.

## Development of the Attachment System

Bowlby (1969) described four stages in the development of the parent–child attachment relationship. In the first stage, the baby's cries are central in gaining attention and support from the caregiver, whose natural response to crying is to draw closer to the baby in order to end an aversive event. Subsequently, the baby's smiles emerge, and these smiles now encourage the parent's proximity in order to maintain a pleasant interaction. In the second stage, babies begin to discriminate among caregivers. This is when they learn they can (or cannot) affect the behavior of others, and can trust (or not trust) them to respond when they signal need. Additionally, babies begin to learn about reciprocity—the concept that in social interactions, partners take turns acting and reacting to each other's actions. By the age of 7 months, babies enter the third stage, where they begin to protest when they are separated from their attachment figure. During this stage (which lasts until approximately 2 years of age), babies are becoming increasingly mobile, and so their chances to move about are substantially increased. As a result, opportunities for exploration and for needing a secure base for that exploration increase significantly. This stage is the crucial one for the formation of attachment that is either secure or insecure (Ainsworth et al., 1978)— an observation that leads me to the work of Mary Ainsworth.

## Mary Ainsworth

Mary Ainsworth was a graduate student at the University of Toronto. One of the faculty members she encountered there was William Blatz, who had devised a theory about children's security (Blatz, 1944). According to this theory, children need to develop a feeling of complete trust in their caregivers; this trust then gives them the courage to explore their environment, to take risks, and, finally, to develop trust in themselves and their own competence. In this way, they move from a state of dependent security to one of independent security. Blatz saw security as a condition characterized by serenity, emerging from belief in one's ability to deal with the future. This ability involves a willingness to accept the consequences of one's decisions, including success and failure, and to develop effective ways of coping with the consequences.

Ainsworth left Toronto in 1950 to accompany her husband to London, England. There, she planned to continue work on the Rorschach test that she had begun in Toronto in collaboration with Bruno Klopfer (Klopfer, Ainsworth, Klopfer, & Holt, 1954, 1956). One Saturday afternoon, however, her attention was drawn to an advertisement in the London *Times* for someone to study the effects of maternal separation under the direction of John Bowlby. Thus began an extraordinarily fruitful collaboration.

In late 1953, Ainsworth went with her husband to Uganda. Inspired by her analyses of Robertson's data in Bowlby's lab, Ainsworth hoped to continue studying children's reactions to separation by taking advantage of the Ugandan custom of sending babies away from their families in order to wean them. However, it turned out that the practice was no longer common, and so she decided to study the development of secure and insecure mother–infant attachment instead (Bretherton, 1992). This interest in different kinds of attachments continued with a move to Johns Hopkins University. There Ainsworth began one of the most famous studies in developmental psychology (Ainsworth et al., 1978), aimed at investigating the nature of mother–child interactions over the first year of life—and, specifically, the precursors of secure and insecure attachment relationships.

Ainsworth hypothesized that mothers who responded immediately to the cries and distress of their babies over the course of the first year of life would have children who, at the age of 1 year, would cry less (and therefore be more securely attached) than those of mothers who were not so responsive. The hypothesis was clearly the opposite of what would be predicted from the learning or reinforcement theory approach to children's social development, which was dominant during the 1960s and 1970s: that mothers who immediately comforted their crying children would reinforce that crying and hence increase the probability that it would occur in the future. This set of alternative hypotheses became the object of considerable debate between Ainsworth and Jacob Gewirtz, with Gewirtz (Gewirtz & Boyd, 1977) arguing that picking up babies would only increase the probability of their crying, and Ainsworth arguing that picking them up or responding to their distress would decrease their crying. Ainsworth won the debate when her observations indicated that babies whose mothers had responded to their crying in the first year of life did indeed cry less than those whose mothers were less responsive. Although responding to children's crying might indeed increase its probability of occurrence later in the course of development, it appeared to operate differently in the first year of life, when a child was more likely to be crying as a result of distress or emotional upset.

## The Strange Situation

Ainsworth had intended to consider the relation between maternal responsiveness to children's distress and children's attachment in the form of reactions to separation from their mothers. However, Baltimore mothers frequently left their babies alone for short periods of time, and so in-home separation did not arouse anxiety on the babies' part. Accordingly, although this was not in the original plan, Ainsworth and Bell (1970) devised a laboratory procedure that they termed the Strange Situation, to see if mothers' responsiveness to crying during the first year of life was a predictor of security or ability to deal with maternal separation in a strange place. It was indeed a predictor: Children of responsive mothers were better able to cope with maternal separation in the laboratory than those of less responsive mothers. Other variables that had been measured at the same time as crying were also predictors of better coping or secure attachment in the Strange Situation, including acceptance and rejection, sensitivity and insensitivity, cooperation and interference, and accessibility and ignoring.

The Strange Situation has become a hugely popular way of studying children's early socioemotional development. Used with children between the ages of 12 and 18 months, it involves a laboratory simulation of how babies and toddlers react when they are separated from their caregivers in a situation that is potentially anxiety-producing. The procedure is made up of seven 3-minute episodes. It begins with the caregiver sitting in a chair while the child plays with toys. A stranger then enters, sits in a chair, talks briefly with the caregiver, and then plays with the child. The caregiver then leaves the room, and the stranger sits in a chair. The caregiver returns (the first reunion episode) and sits in a chair, and the stranger leaves. In the next episode, the caregiver leaves again, so that the child is now completely alone. Then the stranger returns. Finally, the caregiver returns, and the stranger leaves (the second reunion). This whole series of events can be extremely stressful for babies; in fact, the procedure is not infrequently terminated after the first reunion.

Ainsworth had thought that the most informative part of the procedure would be the child's reaction when the caregiver left. What she found, instead, was that the reunion episodes were most revealing, and that they reflected different abilities of caregivers to comfort their children. These different responses to separation and reunion have been repeatedly demonstrated in the multitude of studies that have used the Strange Situation (Cassidy & Shaver, 2016). A majority of babies appear pleased and relieved when their mothers return. Some cry or want to be picked up, but they are soon settled and able to return to play. These are the "secure" children (Type B), who are able to use their caregivers to calm their distress so that they can return to exploration. (Note that the letters used to describe attachment classifications are arbitrary and have no particular meaning.) The remainder of children are insecurely attached, not able to use their caregivers very effectively as sources of comfort. Children with an "anxious–avoidant" attachment pattern (Type A) appear undisturbed by separation, but tend to avoid eye contact with their mothers and will not respond to the mothers' vocalizations or attempts to get close. There is evidence as well that they are physiologically aroused during both separation and reunion, and that their autonomic activity is slow to return to baseline (Sroufe & Waters, 1977). Thus they are indeed upset, but suppress their anger and distress. Babies with an "anxious–resistant" pattern (Type C) protest, cry, and want to be picked up, but are not be able to be comforted by their caregivers. Mothers of Type A babies have been described as intrusive, rejecting, and overstimulating, and those of Type C babies as inconsistent and unresponsive (Belsky, 1999). As a result, presumably, avoidant babies withdraw, whereas resistant babies work hard to get their mothers' attention.

In addition to these three types of attachment, researchers have subsequently identified a fourth—Type D (Main & Solomon, 1990). Type D children are confused or apprehensive about approaching their caregivers during the reunion, and their movements are incomplete or undirected. The Type D or "disorganized" classification has been linked to abusive or other forms of pathological caregiving (Baer & Martinez, 2006). These children are faced with an irresolvable dilemma, given that the caregivers they are evolutionarily driven to seek when they are afraid are also their greatest sources of fear (Main & Hesse, 1990). In this way, disorganized attachment is different from other forms of insecure attachment. Children who exhibit avoidant or resistant responses when they are fearful are exhibiting an appropriate, or "local," response to suboptimal parenting that serves to maximize proximity to their caregivers (Weinfield, Sroufe, Egeland, & Carlson, 2008). Thus an anxious–avoidant child has a caregiver who is not comfortable with displays of emotion, and so the child has learned to minimize those displays. An anxious–resistant child has a caregiver who is inconsistent in responding, and so it becomes necessary for the child to make protection needs known in an insistent way. For the disorganized child, neither such accommodation is possible.

### Attachment in Childhood

The Strange Situation is designed to reflect different ways of dealing with needs for protection in children between 12 and 18 months of age. For older children, researchers have developed other approaches. These include measures such as doll-play scenarios (Bretherton, Bridgeway, & Cassidy, 1990) and family drawings (Kaplan & Main, 1986) designed to reflect the child's expectations with respect to attachment-related issues.

Attachment-related behaviors are altered as children develop. Thus, according to Bowlby (1969), the attachment system changes from one that maintains proximity to the caregiver to one that makes the child aware of the attachment figure's availability. As well, beliefs acquired in the first months of life affect children's subsequent views about achieving security: Children form internal working models or representations of attachment, and these models guide relationships not only with the primary caregiver but with other individuals as well. A secure individual has more constructive representations of other people, more positive expectations for social interactions, a greater understanding of social and emotional events, a more positive self-concept, and a more highly developed conscience than an insecurely attached individual does (Thompson, 2006).

Another outcome of secure attachment is increased compliance with parental directives (see, e.g., Kochanska & Kim, 2012). Recall Stayton et al.'s (1971) proposal that the human species has evolved so that children have a predisposition to comply with parental directives—an important predisposition, because it keeps them safe from danger. Bowlby (1979) talked about parents as "stronger and wiser," and therefore as more likely to be trusted by their children not to make unreasonable requests.

EFFECTS OF INSECURE ATTACHMENT ON PHYSIOLOGICAL INDICES
OF STRESS

Considerable research has focused on the effects of parental lack of responsiveness to distress on events associated with arousal of the hypothalamic–pituitary–adrenocortical (HPA) axis (Koss & Gunnar, 2018). The HPA axis is activated under conditions of stress or anxiety, accompanied by a cascade of neural events involving a large number of brain regions and neurotransmitters. These outcomes enable the individual to take appropriate action in the face of environmental dangers. One of the hormonal accompaniments of activation is cortisol. When activation is too high and too frequent, levels of cortisol are chronically elevated, with negative outcomes such as depression, anxiety, and developmental delay. These effects of high levels of stress continue into middle childhood and beyond. As an example, children reared under conditions of social deprivation in Romanian orphanages but adopted into supportive homes, even when they were very young, still showed higher cortisol levels at 6–12 years of age relative to children without the early deprivation experience. Moreover, when adopted Romanian orphans interacted with their adoptive mothers, their levels of cortisol increased—an indication that these interactions were stressful in spite of a very much improved parenting situation (Gunnar, Morison, Chisholm, & Schuder, 2001; Wismer Fries, Shirtcliff, & Pollak, 2008).

## ■ SOME FEATURES OF ATTACHMENT

The last time I entered "attachment" into a research database, this yielded more than 47,000 entries. I have selected for discussion four topics that have generated considerable research and that are relevant for understanding the protection domain. They have to do with the universality of attachment classifications; the transmission of attachment styles from one generation to the next; the role of temperament in attachment style; and the social and emotional outcomes of different forms of attachment.

### How Universal Are Attachment Classifications?

The answer to the first question seems obvious, given the evolutionary argument that the attachment system allows for survival and reproductive success. The ubiquity of attachment behaviors in various primates is further evidence of universality. In fact, surveys of the literature suggest that attachment behaviors appear in all cultures assessed, although their manifestation is affected by the goals parents have in different societies for their children's behavior toward others.

In a survey of studies of attachment across cultures, van IJzendoorn and Sagi-Schwartz (2008) found not only that all children engage in attachment behaviors directed at adults who serve as their primary caregivers, but that the majority of attachment relationships, regardless of culture, are secure. They also note, however, that there are significant differences in how children react in the Strange Situation. These differences include the number of children in different cultures who fall into various Strange Situation categories. More North German than North American babies, for example, are identified as anxious-avoidant (Grossmann, Grossmann, Spangler, Suess, & Unzner, 1985). This finding has been attributed to the fact that German parents appear to be more likely to encourage independence in their children and to discourage close, clingy contact. In contrast, more Japanese than North American babies are identified as anxious-resistant (Takahashi, 1986). This is presumably because Japanese mothers are more likely to be in constant contact with their children—holding their babies, carrying them, and sleeping with them. Moreover, they rarely leave their children with substitute caregivers (Rothbaum, Weisz, Pott, Miyake, & Morelli, 2000), and this mode of caregiving, not surprisingly, leads to upset in their babies when they are suddenly exposed to the novel experience of separation from their caregivers.

These differences in parenting and outcomes reflect differences in the values and goals parents have for their children in different cultural contexts. Consider the Japanese situation. *Amae,* or a state of total dependence on the mother, is highly desired by Japanese mothers and is considered to be a reflection of maternal love. A healthy sense of *amae* sets the stage for the development of a culturally valued sense of interdependence or communal organization, in which accommodating the needs of others, working toward group goals, and cooperating are of singular importance (Rothbaum et al., 2000; Rothbaum & Trommsdorff, 2007). In contrast, the Western ideal of independence or autonomy influences the patterns of childrearing that characterize so-called "individualist" cultures (Markus & Kitayama, 1991). The resulting differences in attachment-related behaviors, then, reveal some different goals or outcomes that parents hope to achieve. These goals include interdependence versus independence, minimizing versus displaying emotion, and cooperation as opposed to assertiveness (Rothbaum et al., 2000). The different goals, in turn, lead to different ways of expressing attachment-related needs—namely, expressions that work best in one's own cultural context.

## Are Attachment Styles Passed from One Generation to the Next?

A second question has to do with the extent to which attachment styles are transmitted intergenerationally. A number of studies have compared children's attachment status with that of their mothers, with the latter identified by means of the Adult Attachment Interview (AAI; George, Kaplan, & Main, 1985). This interview yields classifications for caregivers that parallel those for children: Adults are classified as "secure-autonomous," "dismissive" (parallel to anxious-avoidant), "preoccupied" (parallel to anxious-resistant), or "unresolved" (parallel to disorganized) on the basis of their responses during an interview to a series of questions probing their mental representations of attachment relationships. Early work indicated that mothers' classifications on the AAI were related to children's attachment status. The finding of such relationships held even when mothers' attachment status was assessed before they had given birth to their children (Fonagy, Steele, & Steele, 1991), and thus before the children's behavior could affect the mothers' ideas about attachment. The finding also held when maternal AAI and child attachment classifications were assessed for mother–child dyads who were not biologically related (Dozier, Stovall, Albus, & Bates, 2001). It would appear, then, that a mother's attachment status is not caused by her child's attachment status; nor is it a reflection of some genetically mediated characteristic they share.

In a meta-analysis of 95 studies assessing the relation between parent representations of attachment and children's attachment status, Verhage et al. (2016) found continuing evidence for intergenerational transmission of attachment, with larger effects for secure-autonomous transmission than for insecure or unresolved transmission. Effect sizes were less but still significant when the sample was high-risk (e.g., a parent was depressed, or was a teenager, or had financial difficulties); when parent and child were not biologically related; and when a child's attachment was assessed at a later age. Interestingly, there was no difference between mothers and fathers in the extent of similarity in attachment styles between themselves and their children.

Of course, transmission of attachment styles or intergenerational continuity is not inevitable. Mental representations of attachment relationships can change, and cycles of harsh parenting can be broken. Among the events that contribute to change are the receipt of positive emotional support from another adult during childhood, participation in therapy, and a supportive and satisfying relationship with a mate (Egeland, Jacobvitz, & Sroufe, 1988). As well, parenting behaviors continue to influence attachment status through adolescence (Allen, Grande, Tan, & Loeb, 2018). Thus maternal support in the form of responsiveness to her adolescent's bids for help predicts a positive change in attachment status (as measured by the AAI). Maternal use of guilt and withdrawal of love is predictive of a negative change in status. Hostile conflict between parents also predicts relative decreases in attachment security, perhaps because it undermines a sense of felt security or because it does not provide a good model for how to resolve relationship problems.

## Are Differences in Attachment Simply Reflections of Differences in Temperament?

The different reactions children have in the Strange Situation could simply be reflections of individual differences in temperament (Kagan, 1982). Thus anxious–avoidant children may also be temperamentally fearless and thus less affected by separation, and anxious–resistant children temperamentally difficult and therefore more affected by separation. However, the fact that an infant may develop different attachment relationships with different caregivers (e.g., a secure attachment to the mother and an insecure one to the father) strongly suggests that temperament does not have a strong causal role to play in determining attachment status (Goossens & van IJzendoorn, 1990).

In a substantial meta-analysis, Groh et al. (2017) found some modest evidence for the role of temperament. Temperament was weakly associated with attachment security, but modestly associated with resistant attachment. Temperament was not significantly associated, however, with either avoidant or disorganized attachment. The link between resistant attachment and temperament, of course, does not rule out the role of parenting in the development of resistant attachments.

The fact that there is minimal evidence for a link between temperament and attachment classification does not mean that there might not be interactions between maternal behavior relevant to attachment and child temperament. Indeed, there is considerable evidence that temperament and parenting in response to distress do interact to affect a variety of child outcomes, such as externalizing and internalizing problems (Bates & Pettit, 2015). As well, temperament does seem to be implicated within each attachment classification (Frodi & Thompson, 1985). Type B babies, for example, range in their reunion behaviors from being quickly able to settle to taking some time to settle, and this makes them closer to avoidant babies in the first case and closer to resistant babies in the second case. Nevertheless, they still satisfy the criteria for secure attachment in a way that avoidant and resistant babies do not.

## Do Securely Attached Children Do Better Socially and Emotionally?

The important question for attachment theory, of course, is how attachment style is related to children's social and emotional outcomes. Do securely attached children do better on various indicants of successful functioning than insecurely attached children? In fact, numerous studies suggest that secure attachment is a significant predictor of a multitude of positive outcomes, such as later successful interactions with parents, peers, and other social partners. In a meta-analysis, Groh et al. (2014) found that avoidant, resistant, and disorganized children showed lower levels of peer competence than those of children who were securely attached. Securely attached children (with attachment assessed at 24 months) have been shown to be involved in less peer conflict than insecurely attached children in first grade (Raikes, Virmani, Thompson, & Hatton, 2013). As well, securely attached children show enhanced problem-solving skills and a less hostile attribution style (i.e., a lesser tendency to assume hostile intent on the part of another child) at 54 months and in first grade, as well as being less lonely (Raikes & Thompson, 2008). In meta-analyses by Fearon, Bakermans-Kranenburg, van IJzendoorn, Lapsley, and Roisman (2010) and by Schneider, Atkinson, and Tardif (2001), securely attached children were found to be more adept at social relationships and at lower risk for both internalizing and externalizing problems. In a review of these and other findings, Thompson (2016) notes that secure attachment has also been linked to a positive self-concept, the development of social cognition and emotion regulation, and fewer behavior problems, as well as to cognitive and language development, exploration and play, curiosity, and math achievement.

Although the evidence for positive outcomes is very strong, it does in fact raise some concerns. Such concerns were reflected in Belsky and Cassidy's (1994) question as to whether there is anything to which attachment security is *not* related. Such concern does suggest that a refinement of the nature of the relation between specific, attachment-related parenting variables and specific child outcomes is in order—a topic to which I now turn.

## ■ MATERNAL RESPONSIVENESS TO DISTRESS VERSUS MATERNAL SENSITIVE RESPONSIVENESS

As noted above, Ainsworth and Bell (1970) identified a number of caregiving behaviors that were associated with behavior in the Strange Situation. In addition to responding to their babies' crying or distress, mothers whose babies were secure were routinely accepting in spite of any frustration or irritation they might have felt. They were sensitively responsive to their babies' signals, interpreting them correctly and responding to them appropriately. They were also careful not to be intrusive or to interfere with their children's activities, and they were accessible rather than ignoring in their reactions. These variables could then, in addition to responsiveness to distress, have been responsible for some of the behaviors seen in the Strange Situation, as well as for some features of the children's subsequent social and emotional development. Indeed, researchers frequently have combined measures of the variables, labeling them as general responsiveness to infant signals (Davidov, 2013).

In reaction to this merging of variables, Goldberg, Grusec, and Jenkins (1999) argued that the notion of caregivers' sensitive responsiveness had been applied too broadly, with a wide variety of parenting behaviors considered to be exemplars of positive attachment-promoting actions. They noted that there had been slippage in some of Bowlby's writings from the original notion of parenting in response to a child's distress or anxiety as a precursor of security, to general responsiveness to infant signals (Bowlby, 1969), but that it was corrected in the second edition (Bowlby, 1982). There Bowlby wrote that what he had in mind when defining attachment behavior was the output of a safety-regulating system designed to reduce the risk of an individual's coming to harm, and in which arousal is experienced as anxiety to be allayed and a sense of security to be increased.

A number of developmentalists have objected to the blurring of attachment's focus. In an analysis of the differences between responsiveness to distress and warmth, for example, MacDonald (1992) noted that maternal warmth is not a ubiquitous feature of parent–child interaction, regardless of culture, whereas caregivers' responsiveness to distress is observed in all cultures. In keeping with the distinction between warmth and mothers' attachment-related behavior, Fox and Davidson (1987) found that the pleasure elicited by a mother's approaching and reaching for her infant was associated with left frontal electroencephalographic (EEG) activation, whereas separation protest was associated with right frontal EEG activation. Belsky and Cassidy (1994) noted that there are different components of the parent–child relationship, including protection, nurturance, play, and control, and that they are related to different outcomes.

Evidence that parental sensitive and responsive reaction to distress needs to be differentiated from other forms of sensitivity and responsiveness comes from other studies. McElwain and Booth-LaForce (2006), for example, found that a mother's sensitivity to her infant's distress at 5 months (the extent to which she responded to her infant's cries, frets, or distress in a consistent and appropriate way) predicted subsequent secure attachment, whereas her sensitivity to nondistressing events (the extent to which she observed and responded to her infant's social gestures, expressions, and signals of nondistress) did not. Davidov and Grusec (2006a) reported that both mothers' and fathers' responsiveness to distress (including emotion- and problem-focused reactions and encouragement of emotion expression), but not their warmth, predicted their children's ability to regulate negative emotions—for example, to recover quickly from upset or distress. In contrast, mothers' warmth, but not their responsiveness to distress, was linked to their children's ability to regulate positive affect—for example, not to become overly excited and, for boys, their greater acceptance by peers. In other studies, early responsiveness to distress has been shown to predict children's subsequent positive social behavior, whereas early responsiveness in play situations has not (Leerkes, Blankson, & O'Brien, 2009). Additionally, although maternal sensitivity to distress and nondistress are modestly positively correlated, they have different antecedents: Mothers who are younger, less well educated, unmarried, and without father involvement are less likely to be sensitive to nondistress cues from their infants, whereas these demographic variables do not predict sensitivity to distress cues (Leerkes, Weaver, & O'Brien, 2012).

The importance of distinguishing between different forms of positive or negative parenting is further underlined by the fact that different positive forms of parenting, as well as negative forms, are either not correlated or only moderately so. These include warmth, responsiveness to distress, calm discussion, proactive teaching, harsh discipline, and acceptance of a child's needs (Davidov & Grusec, 2006a; Landry, Smith, & Swank, 2006, Pettit, Bates, & Dodge, 1997). Finally, mothers who know what their children find comforting do not necessarily know as much about their children's interests and activities (Vinik, Almas, & Grusec, 2011)—another indication of differences in aspects of positive parenting.

## ■ CHILDREN'S COPING, EMPATHY, SYMPATHY, AND PROSOCIAL BEHAVIOR

Children need to learn how to cope with distress and anxiety on their own. Parents help them do this by becoming less protective, applauding successful coping, talking about ways of dealing with distress, and modeling coping behavior. This moves the socialization interaction into the control, guided learning, and group participation domains. These ways of learning are addressed in detail in subsequent chapters. I talk about them here only as they pertain to issues that relate closely to the protection domain—coping, empathy, sympathy, and prosocial behavior that is motivated by empathic arousal. When children are confronted with the distress of others, they experience empathy and sympathy. When they themselves have learned how to cope well, they can turn to assisting others in need (i.e., engaging in prosocial behavior). In the course of such actions, they reduce their own level of empathic distress. When they are not good at coping, however, they may experience personal distress, which leads to a desire to escape the situation rather than improve it.

### Helping Children Deal with Their Own Distress

How do caregivers help children deal successfully with distress on their own? How does development proceed from an understanding that one has a secure base for the provision of safety and comfort, to being able to cope with danger or upset on one's own (to a considerable extent, at least)? Effective caregivers who are successful at helping their children learn to cope are those who initially soothe, hold, and comfort them in frightening situations. As their children grow older, their strategies for providing comfort change. For example, in a study where children were disappointed when they did not get a prize they had been expecting, mothers reacted by shifting their children's attention away from what had happened; by being physically affectionate and saying positive things; and by changing or reframing how the children interpreted the situation, so that it was no longer perceived negatively. Attention refocusing (particularly with preschoolers as opposed to slightly older children), along with cognitive reframing that was done jointly, predicted less sadness at a later point in time (Morris, Silk, Steinberg, Terranova, & Kithakye, 2010; Morris et al., 2011).

Eventually, however, parents need to hand over the responsibility for coping with distress, or at least some of it, to their developing children. Parents who are successful in coaching their children on how to deal with negative affect do so by helping them solve problems, labeling their emotions, and comforting them. Parents who ignore, denigrate, and punish children for expressing negative emotions, or who model counterproductive behavior by becoming distressed themselves, are less successful in teaching them to cope (Criss, Morris, Ponce-Garcia, Cui, & Silk, 2016; Gottman, Katz, & Hooven, 1996; Morris et al., 2011). If a child has lost a prized possession, for example, a successful parent will help the child think of places where he or she might not yet have looked. An unsuccessful one will become upset him or herself or tell the child to be more careful of possessions in the future or not to make such a fuss about the loss. Or if a child is nervous about an upcoming public performance a successful parent will suggest that the child think of something relaxing as a distraction from feelings of anxiousness, whereas an unsuccessful one will tell the child not to be a baby.

## Parents' Knowledge and Children's Coping

Parents who are knowledgeable about their children's thinking with respect to distress are also more likely (with some exceptions noted below) to facilitate their children's coping well with stress. Presumably these parents use their knowledge in order to select a response that is going to be most helpful in the learning process. Vinik et al. (2011), for example, asked young adolescents what would be the best thing their mothers could do when they were worried about preparing for a difficult oral presentation or had lost a favorite possession. Alternatives were presented that included offering assistance, encouraging them to be self-reliant, expressing sympathy, and suggesting diversions such as going for a special food treat. Mothers were asked to say how they thought their adolescents would rate each of these ways of responding. The closer mothers' ratings were to those of their children, the better the adolescents' performance on a measure of positive coping that included seeking social support (e.g., asking a friend for help when needed) and being self-reliant and engaging in problem solving (e.g., deciding on a way to deal with the problem and doing it). This relation between mothers' knowledge and adolescents' coping held only for children who rated themselves as more likely to be upset by a variety of stressful events, presumably because their mothers had more opportunity to witness their distress and therefore had more opportunities to learn about what were successful parenting strategies.

The finding by Vinik et al. does not mean that mothers necessarily responded to their children's upset by providing them with the form of comfort they liked best. It does mean that they knew enough about their children in the protection domain to be able to teach and achieve successful outcomes. Relatedly, a longitudinal study (Sherman, Grusec, & Almas, 2017) found that mothers who said they were dissatisfied with some aspect of their adolescents' behavior, and who were more knowledgeable about their adolescents' preferred coping strategies, had children who coped better at a 2-year follow-up. Sherman et al. suggested that knowledgeable mothers who find their children's behavior less than positive use that knowledge to improve coping ability.

Knowledge and positive outcomes are not always related, however. Kiel and Buss (2011) assessed the ability of mothers of fearful toddlers to predict how their toddlers would react to novel events, such as an adult dressed as a clown. Over a 3-year period, they found that the more accurate mothers were, the *more* socially withdrawn their children were. This relation was mediated by mothers' overprotectiveness in the form of high levels of supporting and comforting in response to their children's reactions to the novel events. Thus knowledgeable mothers of fearful children seemed to use their knowledge to be overly protective, with negative consequences for their children's emotional outcomes. This finding raises the issue, then, of how much support parents should provide as they teach their children to be able to cope with stress. Here I turn to a discussion of parenting that is just good enough and not overly nice.

## "Good-Enough" and "Not-Too-Nice" Parenting

The British psychoanalyst Donald Winnicott (1953) wrote about the "good-enough" mother who helps her child become independent by starting off with almost complete adaptation to her infant's needs, but who adapts less and less as time goes on, in keeping with her child's ability to deal with or compensate for her apparent failure. In a similar vein, Bates and Pettit (2015) write about "not-too-nice" parenting, in which the parent is not too quick to offer support. Bates and Pettit begin with the frequently replicated finding that children with a fearful temperament are more likely to have anxiety problems at a later time. However, they also note a pattern whereby fearful children are less likely to have such problems when parents are more challenging, intrusive, and frustrating (but not denigrating), as opposed to being highly supportive or comforting. With experience, the children of these parents become more skilled at handling novel situations, and parents help the process by encouraging mastery of initially fearful situations. Bates and Pettit suggest that one way in which parental protectiveness has harmful effects is through a process of negative reinforcement: Parents eventually give in to their children's display of distress to end an unpleasant event, and so the children's problem behavior is reinforced. As these experiences accumulate, the children lag in ability to self-regulate and in social skills—a deficit that provides further reasons for anxiety. Bates and Pettit propose that a combination of warmth and high control (i.e., parental solicitousness) is responsible for these negative outcomes.

Further evidence for the usefulness of a "not-so-nice" parenting strategy, particularly with timid children, comes from a number of studies. Rubin, Burgess, and Hastings (2002), for example, found that timid children whose mothers were particularly solicitous and comforting displayed greater social wariness than children whose mothers were less solicitous, and Degnan, Henderson, Fox, and Rubin (2008) further showed that maternal solicitous behavior is a factor involved in the maintenance of social wariness from preschool to childhood. In a longitudinal study, Hastings, Kahle, and Nuselovici (2014) assessed not only mothers' overprotection, but also their preschoolers' physiological ability to regulate cardiac activity, and therefore to be able to diminish their reactivity to social situations. Children who were socially wary had anxiety problems and fewer social skills when these were measured 5 years later, but only when both maternal overprotection and lessened ability to decrease acute arousal states were present.

SUMMARY■ ■ ■ ■ ■ ■ ■ ■ ■ ■ ■ ■ ■ ■ ■ ■ ■ ■ ■ ■ ■ ■ ■ ■ ■ ■ ■ ■ ■ ■ ■ ■

Parents build on an early base of protective parenting by modeling and teaching effective coping behaviors, including problem solving and accurate identification of emotions. They do not ignore or punish the display of emotions, and they do not deny their legitimacy. They do not become upset themselves. Parents who know how their children think with respect to protection-related events can use this knowledge to improve coping skills. However, knowledge can be problematic if it leads to overly solicitous behavior. Much of the research on children's coping emphasizes the dangers of overprotection—a condition particularly likely to arise when children are timid or anxiety-prone. Presumably, it is more challenging for parents of timid children to engage in "good-enough" or "not-too-nice" parenting than it is for those of children who are less anxious about their environment. Nevertheless, the latter still need guidance in how to deal with stress; this guidance comes about through modeling of stress-reducing actions, as well as discussions of how to deal with challenging situations.

## Empathy, Sympathy, Personal Distress, and Concern for Others

Successfully socialized children not only respond appropriately to their own distress, but also respond to the distress of others. This is because the observation of distress in another person activates some of the same neural substrates that are activated when observers themselves are feeling the same emotion (Decety, 2011). This empathic response—experiencing the same emotion as another—can then become a motivator of prosocial behavior that is intended to reduce one's own unpleasant feelings as well as those of the person (or animal) experiencing the distress. Older children who can differentiate between the self and others, who have improved perspective-taking skills, and who have been encouraged by parenting practices that include other-oriented reasoning, manifest their arousal as sympathy—a feeling of concern for a distressed other, but not an actual sharing of their emotion (Eisenberg et al., 2006; Malti, Dys, Colasante, & Peplak, 2018). Sympathy, again, is a motivator of helpful action.

Empathy and sympathy for the plight of others facilitate prosocial behavior, but especially so when individuals can cope successfully with their own feelings of distress. When levels of empathy and sympathy become too great (i.e., when coping skills are not well developed), feelings of personal distress emerge (Batson, Futz, & Schoenrade, 1987; Eisenberg et al., 2006). Not being able to deal with a negative or highly arousing experience can result in attempts to avoid others who are experiencing a negative state rather than trying to assist them. Whereas empathy and sympathy are frequently related to prosocial behavior, personal distress is not. Thus higher levels of skin conductance and increases in heart rate, indicants of distress, are predictive of lower levels of children's responsiveness to distress in others (Eisenberg et al., 2006).

An example of how parenting can foster either prosocial behavior that is motivated by sympathetic concern or anxious behavior that is motivated by personal distress is provided by Eisenberg, Spinrad, Taylor, and Liew (2017). Eisenberg et al. observed mothers and toddlers interacting in a stressful situation. There were differences in how mothers responded, with some being supportive by distracting their children's attention from the distressing situation or by helping them to solve the stress-producing problem. Others were less supportive. Toddlers were then exposed to an adult female who had "accidentally" hurt herself. Children of supportive mothers reacted to the adult by engaging in comforting actions such as patting the adult or attracting their mothers' attention. Children with mothers who were less supportive, on the other hand, tended to display personal distress by going to their mothers, touching their mothers, holding their arms out to be picked up, or burying their heads in the mothers' lap. Thus they were much less able to reach out to help someone in need of support.

The relations among mothers' supportive behavior, children's ability to cope with distress, and older children's prosocial behavior was examined in a recent study (Kil, Grusec, & Chaparro, 2018). In this study, the mothers of young adolescents were asked how likely they would be to talk to their children about moderately distressing events, such as having to give a presentation or losing a prized object. Their children's ability to cope was assessed, along with teachers' ratings of how helpful the children were in the classroom. Results indicated that coping mediated between mothers' disclosure and children's classroom behavior. Thus mothers who provided opportunities for discussion about how to deal with distress, and for whom this resulted in increases in their children's ability to cope, were more likely to have children who responded to distress in others.

■ CONCLUSION

In the protection domain, a child develops a positive relationship with a caregiver whom the child knows he or she can rely on for care in unsafe or anxiety-producing situations. A key component in the relationship is the development of trust—trust that the caregiver will be there when and if needed, as well as trust that demands that are made will be reasonable and in the child's best interests. Socialization in the protection domain begins at birth but continues throughout the course of development. The present chapter has focused on the protection relationship as one of the two bases of successful socialization. The second base is reciprocity, the topic of Chapter 4.

**CHAPTER 1 SCENARIOS REVISITED**

In Chapter 1, in my introduction to the five domains of socialization, I have described two situations involving a child who was experiencing distress in the protection domain. Those vignettes are reproduced in Box 3.1, along with three possible reactions a parent might have in each of them. In light of the research described in the present chapter, one reaction is better than the other two in each situation.

In the first vignette, a young boy is afraid of dogs. In Alternative A, his father dismisses and denigrates his fears—not a reaction conducive to learning how to cope. In Alternative B the father is overprotective. This, too, is not an optimal response. Alternative C, where the father engages in good-enough or not-so-nice parenting by gently urging exposure to the dog, would seem the preferable way to deal with the problem.

The second vignette involves a 12-year-old who has had a fight with her best friend. In Alternative A, her mother dismisses her distress, which is not the best approach. In Alternative C, the mother herself becomes distressed—again, not optimal. Alternative B seems the best approach: comforting her daughter and also suggesting a positive way of improving the situation.

**BOX 3.1.** Scenarios from the Protection Domain

*Chris (6 years old) is invited to a neighbor's house to see their new dog. Chris hasn't had much experience with dogs, and he says he's afraid and doesn't want to go.*

A. Dad says, "Don't be silly. Big boys like you shouldn't be afraid of dogs."

B. Dad says, "I understand. You don't need to go."

C. Dad says, "I understand. You haven't been around dogs much, and it certainly isn't a good idea to pat a strange dog. Why don't we go next door to see the new dog, and we'll play with him together?"

*Janice (12 years old) comes home from school looking very sad and immediately goes to her room. Her mother asks if anything is wrong. Janice says that she has just had a fight with her best friend and is afraid they will never be friends again.*

A. Mom says, "Don't worry. You have lots of friends."

B. Mom says, "Why don't we talk about what happened and see if there's a way for the two of you to get back together? Maybe she's just as unhappy about the fight as you are."

C. Mom says, "That's so sad. I remember when my best friend and I had a fight, and it wasn't a pleasant time."

# CHAPTER 4

# The Reciprocity Domain

*Compliance with Reasonable Requests*

H umans have evolved to reciprocate favors—a characteristic that, as protection does, contributes to their survival and reproductive success (Trevarthen, Kokkinski, & Flamenghi, 1999). As a result, they exhibit a strong tendency to assist others and to want to receive benefits from those others in return. Although helping others who are not biologically related does not directly facilitate individuals' reproductive success, it does contribute to their survival, and therefore ultimately to their successful reproduction. An important feature of reciprocity is knowing when one has been treated unfairly, particularly by those who are not genetically related. And so it has been proposed that people have been endowed with a "cheater mechanism," which makes them sensitive to times when they provide benefits to others but do not receive benefits in exchange. This ability to detect cheating does not depend on past experience, and it appears to develop at an early age and across cultures (Cosmides & Tooby, 1992). Evidence for such a cheater mechanism comes from the observation that "source memory"—memory for the context in which a face has been encountered—is consistently better for the faces of cheaters than for other types of faces (Buchner, Bell, Mehl, & Musch, 2009).

The universal tendency to reciprocate favors is also present in the socialization process. Thus socialization in the reciprocity domain involves a mutual exchange of favors between parent and child. In

65

short, when caregivers go along with the reasonable requests, wishes, desires, or needs of their children, their children are more likely to go along with or comply with reasonable requests from the caregivers. Socializing agents themselves are compliant, and this compliance, in turn, elicits compliance from their children. Notable in this domain is that parents and children have equal power in the interaction.

In the reciprocity domain, caregivers do not teach specific values. The reciprocity domain is similar in this way to the protection domain, where the focus is on developing a positive relationship that forms the basis for subsequent teaching. In the protection domain, children are motivated to act in accord with societal values, because they trust their parents to recommend actions that are in their own best interests. In the reciprocity domain, children are motivated to act in accord with parents' values, because they see themselves as part of an interacting dyad whose members have mutually compatible goals. What happens in the reciprocity domain contributes to the development of a relationship that underpins and determines the effectiveness of direct teaching that occurs in the other three domains. In the control domain, parents use discipline and explanation to modify antisocial behavior or promote prosocial behavior. In the guided learning domain, they talk with their children about the nature of acceptable behavior. And in the group participation domain, they manage the environment so that their children are exposed to positive social behavior. In contrast, in the reciprocity domain, they lay the groundwork that makes specific teaching effective; the emphasis in this domain is on interaction and exchange.


## ■ PARENT–CHILD INTERACTION

Talking about exchanges and reciprocity in relationships is not always easy for socialization theorists. There is a strong tendency to think in terms of the parent as the causal agent or leader who guides and maintains behavior. Thus researchers frequently need to be reminded that socialization is a bidirectional process (Bell & Harper, 1977; Kuczynski & De Mol, 2015), with parents' actions not only affecting children's actions, but vice versa. Beyond this simple model, however, is a more complex one that focuses on the back-and-forth exchanges or interactions between parent and child—in which each partner influences, and each is affected by, the actions of the other.

## Interaction Theory

Children and socializing agents not only act in a relationship, but react as well. Interaction theory moves beyond a focus on the child's impact on the parent by pointing out that socializing agents and children are involved in extended interchanges or chains of responses, not just one single exchange. Thus a child not only acts but reacts in a relationship (Cairns, 1979), with this reaction determined not just by an immediately preceding response, but, additionally and importantly, by earlier actions and their results. The notion of interaction is not a novel one, appearing in work by early developmental psychologists. James Mark Baldwin (1906), for example, noted that children are embedded in a social network, and that their personalities undergo continuous modification as a result of the reactions or feedback they receive from other people in the network. Somewhat more recently, the developmental psychologist James Youniss (1980) pointed out that "actions can have reliable meaning only when they are understood as reciprocal to the actions of other persons" (p. 234).

Maccoby and Martin (1983), in an influential review of the socialization literature, suggested that one way of viewing social interactions is to see them as scripts. One of the earliest scripts shared by infants and adults is that of mutual imitation, where caregiver and child engage in a simple exchange (such as tongue protrusion) that involves turn taking and that requires a straightforward reaction to each other's actions (Meltzoff & Moore, 1977). In these scripts, the caregiver not only reflects back the child's behavior, but also produces a predictable form of his or her own behavior. Exchanges move into more sophisticated territory as the child learns new and more complex scripts, involving a more elaborated set of expectations. Children are very invested in these scripts and can become distressed when there is disruption in an expected interaction. An example of this distress in infancy is the "still-face" demonstration (Tronick, Als, Adamson, Wise, & Brazelton, 1978). In this demonstration, mothers are first instructed to play normally with their infants. Then they are instructed to stop playing and to keep a poker or still face, looking at their infants but not smiling, talking, or touching the infants. Infants' reactions to this stilling include unhappiness and distress; they look sad or angry, scan their surroundings, reach out to be picked up, twist and turn in their seats, hiccup, spit up, and turn their attention to inanimate toys as a way of coping with their distress at their mothers' failure to engage in an expected exchange (Gianino & Tronick, 1988).

## Control Systems Theory

Another analysis of parent–child interaction patterns comes from control systems theory (Bell & Harper, 1977). In this analysis, each member of a dyad is seen as establishing an acceptable range for the appropriateness, strength, and frequency of behavior displayed by the other member. When the range becomes unacceptable—either too great or too small—some action has to be taken to restore equilibrium. When, for example, children behave badly, parents will take some action to return behavior to an acceptable level. Or when children are not interacting, parents may work to encourage a higher level of interaction. Similarly, when parents are nonresponsive, children will work to increase the level of caregiver responsiveness; when parents exert too much control, children will take steps to dampen that level of control. When the efforts of either member of the dyad are not successful in moving the interaction back to an acceptable level, participants will be driven apart, and the relationship will be impaired. Note, of course, that different dyads have different ideas about what is an acceptable range for a given behavior. Thus some parents and children have greater tolerance for particular behaviors than do other parents and children.

## ■ RECIPROCITY AND READINESS TO BE SOCIALIZED

Maccoby and Martin (1983) extended ideas associated with parent–child interaction to the realm of compliance, asking how agents of socialization might encourage their children's willingness to cooperate with requests and directives. Ideas associated with parent–child interaction and exchange provided some new clues for how this might be achieved.

Children differ in how easily they respond to a parent's request for compliance. Some are reasonably willing to stop arguing with a sibling, or take out the garbage, or share a toy, or make their beds, or clean the kitty litter box. Others are less willing to do so. Maccoby and Martin suggested that children's willingness to engage in behavior exchange is a factor that can mediate between a parent's request or pressure for change and the child's ready willingness to take a receptive stance toward the request. What makes a child receptive? What sort of parenting makes interactions smooth and cooperative rather than confrontational? How can escalation of conflict be avoided as the child fails to comply and the parent becomes angry, frustrated, and increasingly pressuring, with the resulting impairment of a positive and peaceful relationship? The answer, they proposed, could be found in whether or not parent and child had developed a system of mutual exchange of compliant behavior. They found that when caregivers complied with children's reasonable requests and bids for interaction, children would, in turn, comply with the caregivers' reasonable requests. Because compliance is part of a chain of reactions, it leads to "receptive compliance" (which is willingly given) rather than to "situational compliance" (which is forced). I consider these two forms of compliance in turn.

## Receptive and Situational Compliance

### Receptive Compliance

Early evidence for the socialization of receptive compliance was provided by attachment theorists. In a study of the relation between attachment and compliance, for example, Matas, Arend, and Sroufe (1978) found that children who were securely attached at 18 months were more compliant with their mothers' various requests when the dyads were observed in a laboratory setting 6 months later. Matas et al. argued that attachment style is the mediator between a mother's sensitive responsiveness and a child's cooperative compliance, with compliance a reflection of trust in the mother as a secure base. Maccoby and Martin (1983), however, pointed out that the wide variety of parenting actions related to secure attachment includes sensitivity, cooperation, acceptance, accessibility, sociability, and displays of positive affect—all features of positive dyadic exchanges. They argued that some of these actions may be directly responsible for children's compliance, and that there is therefore no need to call on attachment style as a mediator or explanation.

Early research that had looked directly at the relation between a parent's compliance and sensitivity to a child's needs and state supported Maccoby and Martin's argument. Stayton et al. (1971), for example, found that maternal sensitivity, cooperation, and acceptance were directly related to 12-month-old children's compliance. In another study (Schaffer & Crook, 1980), mothers were asked to make sure that their children played with each of a number of different toys with which they had been provided. Mothers were most successful at gaining compliance when they adjusted their interventions to the children's immediately preceding state. Thus, when children were asked to touch a toy, mothers were more successful if their children were oriented to the toy, and when children were asked to play with a toy, mothers were more successful if their children were actually touching it. In essence, then, mothers who were sensitive to their children's current attentional state, and who matched their own actions to that state, were more effective at gaining compliance than were those who issued directions or requests that did not fit with the children's current orientation. Among these features of sensitivity would be a mother's own willingness to comply with her child's requests.

Receptive compliance happens when children do not feel forced to obey. Associated with their feeling of freedom of choice, and hence with the presence of a cooperative and receptive style, are the caregiver's sensitivity, cooperation, acceptance, emotional bonding, fostering of trust, high levels of playful behavior in an emotionally positive context, and frequent joint task-related activity. Maccoby and Martin (1983) described the outcome of these features of parenting in the following way:

> Parents who are themselves cooperative with their children's needs tend to have children who are cooperative with theirs; parents who are trustworthy tend to have children who trust them and thus cooperate with them; parents who themselves legitimize their children's needs and desires tend to have children who treat their parents' needs and desires as legitimate as well. (p. 68)

### Situational Compliance

In contrast to receptive compliance, situational compliance implies coercion on the part of the socializing agent. Although direct demands and threats elicit immediate compliance, a great many studies indicate that such compliance is not long-lasting and does not generalize to other situations. Thus, for example, strict parenting that is not responsive to the needs and wishes of the child undermines willingness to go along with the requests of others in the absence of surveillance. Although it may produce immediate compliance, it is ineffective in promoting compliance that endures beyond the immediate context (Baumrind, 2012).

## Parental Compliance and the Development of Children's Compliance

To see if maternal cooperation and compliance was a precursor of children's compliance, Parpal and Maccoby (1985) compared 3- to

4-year-old children's compliance across three experimental conditions. In the first condition, mothers were instructed to fill out questionnaires while their children played with toys by themselves. In the second condition, mothers were asked to play with their children and the toys as they normally would. In a short session a week previously, mothers in the third condition had been trained how to play responsively with their children—including describing and imitating their children's behavior; complying with their children's suggestions and directives; and eliminating questions, commands, and criticisms during play activity. At the experimental session, these mothers were asked to play with their children in the way they had been trained to in the previous week. After 15 minutes, all mothers were asked to stop what they were doing—filling out questionnaires or playing with their children—and to get their children to put away the toys with which they had been playing. The researchers found that children whose mothers had been trained to play responsively were significantly more likely to comply with their request. In essence, these children demonstrated an increased readiness to accept the influence attempts of their mothers when their mothers had first shown a willingness to accept *their* influence attempts. The data also suggested that training in responsiveness was especially effective for children who were rated as difficult and noncompliant by their mothers and their teachers.

One explanation Parpal and Maccoby offered for the increase in children's compliance was that responsive play by mothers puts children into a better frame of mind, and that being in a good mood makes people more likely to respond to others in a positive social way (Underwood, Froming, & Moore, 1977). To test this hypothesis, Lay, Waters, and Park (1989) had mothers and preschoolers play together as they had in the Parpal and Maccoby study, with mothers instructed either to be responsive in their play or to play normally. Children were then shown cartoon drawings of happy, sad, and neutral faces and asked to say which face felt most like them. Those in the responsive play condition reported feeling happier than those in the normal play condition, as the researchers had predicted. In a second study, Lay et al. assessed the causal link between emotion and compliance by manipulating children's emotions. They did this by asking children to think of something that made them feel happy, good, excited, upset, scared, or angry. Their mothers were then told to ask that their children put toys away. Children who had been asked to imagine themselves in a positive mood complied more than those who were in a negative mood. Lay et al. concluded that positive interactions between adult and child create a positive affective context, and that this positive affect is instrumental in promoting compliance and the development of positive social behavior.

## Reciprocity versus Control

In talking about the importance of positive affect, Maccoby (1983) commented on the almost exclusive emphasis on negative emotions by socialization researchers—an emphasis that included attachment theory with its focus on distress, as well as research on discipline with its focus on guilt. Maccoby argued that whereas negative affect is an important aspect of the socialization process, positive events are also important. Thus a child whose caregiver has been responsive in the first 18 or so months of life, when parental demands are less frequent, "has put assets into the socialization bank—assets that can be drawn upon when the child has developed to the point when socialization pressures are necessary" (p. 363). Affection or responsiveness in the control domain involves making children obey because they fear losing love or emotional support. Reciprocity, in contrast, offers a positive role for the parent–child relationship. Thus a responsive and positively affective stance on the parent's part promotes the child's willingness to pay attention and to become interested in and cooperative with parental suggestions. In this way, power-assertive modes of interaction that require a winner, a loser, a compromise, or a standoff become unnecessary for successful socialization. Reciprocity does not entail conflict, because caregiver and child share the same goals; in the reciprocity domain there is no coercion, but only a willing exchange.

## Training Mothers to Be More Compliant, and Long-Term Effects

In Parpal and Maccoby's (1985) study, maternal compliance training was of very short duration, and the effects were evaluated immediately after the training. More recent studies have used longer training periods and assessed effects over a longer period of time. Kochanska, Kim, Boldt, and Nordling (2013), for example, employed a 10-week training program in which mothers of toddlers practiced attending to what their children were doing; following their children's lead; being positive and rewarding; and not asking questions, issuing commands or suggestions, teaching, or making critical/negative comments. After this extensive training, their children's compliance in a laboratory test was compared with that of toddlers whose mothers had been instructed over the same 10-week period to play as they usually did. In an immediate follow-up, both groups were more compliant than a control group with no play experience. However, 6 months later, children in the group where mothers had been trained to follow their children's lead were now more compliant than those who played as usual. It seems, then, that one very useful way of increasing children's enduring compliance is to provide training for parents in how to let their children lead social interactions.

## ■ MUTUAL RECIPROCITY AND SYNCHRONY

The idea of socialization as a process of incorporating a child into a system of reciprocity, rather than as an imposition of an authority figure's wishes on the child, has been developed by a number of researchers. Building on the work of Maccoby and her colleagues, Kochanska (1997) proposed that mutually responsive or communal relationships promote the adoption of positive social behavior by the child as the parent acts responsively to the child's needs. When such mutually responsive relationships do not develop, the dyad members can become adversaries: Because they have different goals from their children, parents must therefore apply pressure in order to gain compliance. One consequence of mutual responsiveness, then, is a reduced need for the use of power-assertive interventions or coercion.

### Features of a Reciprocal Relationship

What exactly does it mean to be involved in a reciprocal relationship? What sort of behavior would one expect to see on the part of caregiver and child? Kochanska (1997) describes a mutually responsive orientation that reflects a close, mutually binding, cooperative, and affectively positive relationship. Kochanska identified two components of such a relationship: mutual cooperation or responsiveness, and shared positive affect involving smoothly flowing interactions that provide positive emotional experiences for both dyad members. In early studies, Kochanska and colleagues examined each member of the dyad separately to arrive at a final measure of reciprocity, Later work has measured dyadic quality explicitly. This dyadic quality consists of several dimensions. The first dimension is that of "coordinated routines," including smooth interactions and signs of shared expectations about what comes next. As examples, at 7 months, babies anticipate routines by opening their mouths as food is delivered on a spoon; at 15 months, they lift their chins so that their bibs can be put on; and at 25 months, they participate in choosing food items and may open food containers while mothers hold a paper towel in anticipation of a minor spill. Kochanska's second dimension is "mutual cooperation," involving satisfactory resolution of conflicts and openness to each other's influence. Next is "harmonious communication," in the form of effortless exchanges conducted in a back-and-forth manner. The final dimension is "emotional ambiance," or expressions of affection and pleasure in each other's company (Aksan, Kochanska, & Ortmann, 2006).

"Synchrony" is a term that has been used by other researchers to describe these harmonious parent–child interactions (e.g., Feldman, 2012; Harrist & Waugh, 2002). Five components of synchrony are outlined by Lindsey, Cremeens, Colwell, and Caldera (2009). The first is "dyadic reciprocity," involving contingent exchanges such as sharing the same focus of attention and mirroring each other's emotional state. The second and third involve the extent to which positive and negative emotions are shared, including smiles, laugher, sadness, and anger. "Mutual initiation" (i.e., the balance between a parent's and child's attempts to influence each other's behavior) and "mutual compliance" are the final two components. Synchrony and reciprocity, then, overlap considerably in their emphasis on coordination, cooperation, and shared affect.

## Outcomes of Mutually Regulated or Synchronous Interactions

A great many positive outcomes are associated with mutually regulated or synchronous parent–child interactions, beyond immediate compliance. These include secure attachment relationships (Isabella & Belsky, 1991), better self-regulation (Lindsey et al., 2009), peer competence (Harrist, Petit, Dodge, & Bates, 1994; Lindsey, Cremeens, & Caldera, 2010a), positive self-esteem and prosocial behavior (Lindsey et al., 2010a), and receptive compliance and future conscience development (Kochanska, Aksan, Prisco, & Adams, 2008). Synchrony is negatively correlated with externalizing problems, but only when adults and children are above average in the positive nature of their interaction (Deater-Deckard, Atzaba-Poria, & Pike, 2004)—a finding supporting the idea that mutuality works better in a context of warmth.

## Are the Effects of Synchrony General or Specific?

One important question emerging from this wide variety of outcomes is
whether mutual regulation is a global characteristic of the parent–child
relationship that accounts for a whole variety of benefits, or whether
some or each of its components may be a predictor of different aspects
of successful socialization. In Chapter 3, I have noted that different
forms of responsiveness (such as warmth, responsiveness to distress,
acceptance, and rejection) are associated with different child outcomes.
The discussion in Chapter 3 is relevant here as well. Thus some parts of
the synchronous relationship may be associated more closely with some
positive child outcomes than with others. Isabella and Belsky (1991),
for example, found that different aspects of synchrony were related to
mother–infant attachment status: anxious-avoidant babies had mothers who were intrusive and overstimulating, whereas anxious-resistant
babies had mothers who were underinvolved and inconsistent. Bornstein and Tamis-LeMonda (1997) found that mothers' responsiveness to
children's vocalizations was related to language development but not to
quality of play, whereas responsiveness to play was related to the quality
of children's play but not to language development.

## Characteristics of Children and Caregivers That Affect Synchronous Interaction

Children and caregivers bring different characteristics to their interaction, some of which may facilitate and some of which may inhibit that
interaction. In the case of children, for example, studies have shown
that siblings who are genetically similar tend to have relationships with
their mothers that are more similar in levels of mutuality, whereas
this is not the case for unrelated adopted siblings (Deater-Deckard &
O'Connor, 2000; Deater-Deckard & Petrill, 2004). This result speaks
to the roles that differences in inborn temperament, such as fearfulness, outgoingness, or positive affectivity, might play in parent–child
interaction. With respect to caregivers, Feldman et al. (2009) note that
anxiety and depression both affect the temporal pattern of early parent–
child interactions; intrusive maternal behavior is associated with anxiety, and minimal mothering with depression. Stress is another variable that contributes to problematic interactions (Im-Bolter, Anam, &
Cohen, 2015). No doubt it is a factor in the finding that mothers who
are married and who have fewer children—and who, presumably, are

therefore less stressed—engage in greater levels of child-oriented play (Kochanska et al., 2013). Yet another determinant of levels of synchronous interaction is parent gender: Fathers do not differ from mothers in their caregiving behavior, but they are more directive in their play interactions (Lindsey, Cremeens, & Caldera, 2010b).

## ■ SYNCHRONY VERSUS PARENTAL RESPONSIVENESS TO CHILD REQUESTS

Are synchrony and responding to children's reasonable requests the same thing? In the former case, parent and child are involved in a happy back-and-forth exchange where each accommodates the expectations of the other. In the latter case, a parent is, to use Maccoby's (1983) analogy, putting assets into the socialization bank by complying with the child's reasonable requests. Do the two approaches have different effects on children's compliance? The results of a recent study (Davidov, Tuvia, Polacheck, & Grusec, 2018), comparing the effects of a child's and parent's having joint leadership in interactions (synchrony) and the parent's allowing the child to lead the interaction (parental responsiveness to the child's requests), suggest that the two approaches may not be identical in their effects.

In this study, 6- to 8-year-old children and their mothers were observed during a 15-minute play session, and the extent to which mothers followed their children's lead during play and the extent to which they shared the lead during play were both assessed. Following the child's lead included mothers' allowing their children to choose activities and determine the progression of play, cooperating with the children's ideas and suggestions, being engaged and interested, and repeating and elaborating on their children's ideas, but refraining from making their own suggestions or directives. Sharing the lead reflected the extent to which a mother and child led the interaction together, as equals, and in a mutual and balanced manner. After the play session, mothers were asked to make three requests of their children—place a magazine on a shelf in the playroom, draw a picture on a blackboard, and throw a piece of paper into the trash. Ratings were also made by teachers of the children's concern and consideration for others in the classroom.

The extent to which children had been allowed to lead the interaction was a positive predictor of their immediate compliance, but, similar to the findings of Parpal and Maccoby (1985), only in the case of children who were rated as difficult by their mothers. In contrast, the extent to which the lead was joint, or the play synchronous, was a predictor of immediate compliance for all children, regardless of how difficult their mothers said they were. One possible explanation for this finding is that difficult children are put into a positive state of mind when they are allowed to direct play, and this makes them more amenable to a request for compliance. Easy children, on the other hand, are generally cooperative without a need for priming. With respect to sharing the lead, compliance may simply be part of an ongoing reciprocal and positive exchange between parent and child. An even larger difference between the two groups was observed when teachers were asked to rate the children's rule-following and cooperative behavior in the classroom; both types of behavior were associated with the extent to which children were allowed to take the lead, but not with the extent to which children shared the lead with their mothers. A possible explanation here is that in the case of following the children's lead, mothers may have been providing a model of consideration for others' wishes, with this modeling helping children become more cooperative in interactions with others outside the home. Perhaps, in the case of sharing the lead, these parents were providing practice in useful social skills such as how to interact with others in a relationship that involves pleasant ongoing and mutual exchanges.

## Maternal Depression and Sharing the Lead

The suggestion that sharing the lead promotes social competence is supported in an analysis of the interaction between depressed mothers and their children by Yan and Dix (2014). They describe a cascade of events beginning in the preschool years and extending into grade school, with lower levels of synchronous interaction eventually leading to deficiencies in social interactions with peers. Yan and Dix found that the children of depressed mothers became more withdrawn over time, with increases in withdrawal predicting declines in positive mutuality in these mother–child dyads. This decline, in turn, was associated with children's poor school adjustment as measured by academic achievement and problems in social competence. Yan and Dix suggest that depressive symptoms in mothers promote inhibition and withdrawal in their children, so that these dyads are less likely to engage in activities such as play and other forms of exchange that promote social competence.

Because their mothers are nonresponsive or intrusive, these children do not develop a sense of self-efficacy or a feeling that they can influence the actions of others, and they thereby lose out on the opportunity to learn basic social competencies. Instead, they acquire maladaptive ways of dealing with emotional interactions by avoiding others and developing negative expectations about social encounters.

## SUMMARY■ ■ ■ ■ ■ ■ ■ ■ ■ ■ ■ ■ ■ ■ ■ ■ ■ ■ ■ ■ ■ ■ ■ ■ ■ ■ ■ ■ ■ ■ ■ ■ ■ ■ ■ ■

Two approaches to the study of reciprocity have been taken by researchers. The first involves a situation in which parents invest in future compliance by setting examples of responsive compliance, particularly when children are young and parental demands are less frequent. This does not mean, however, that children who are older do not respond to parental compliance, particularly if they are difficult children. The second approach involves a back-and-forth exchange in which parents and children take turns in leading the interaction, which includes positive affect on both their parts. What evidence there is suggests that the two events have somewhat different outcomes. Practice in synchronous interactions no doubt teaches social skills and adeptness at interacting with others, as well as increasing willingness to go along with the wishes of others. Having parents who comply with reasonable requests builds up a store of good will that promotes later cooperation. Both parental compliance and synchronous interaction put children into a positive mood state, and this may make them more likely to be compliant. Parental compliance may also provide a model of considerate behavior that children emulate.

## ■ MOVING BEYOND PLAY: HEALTHY NUTRITION AND TECHNOLOGY USE

Research on reciprocity has focused largely on play situations. But parents and children interact in many other settings as well. One such setting is mealtime, where the goal is to teach children healthy eating habits. Given that the learning of such habits is a central concern for parents, diet can become a serious source of parent–child conflict. Bringing ideas about reciprocity and bidirectionality to bear on the topic, Walton, Kuczynski, Haycraft, Breen, and Haines (2017) have argued that children's "picky eating" should be reconceptualized as a reflection of their agency with respect to eating preferences, rather than as an issue of parental control, and that this approach is best addressed within a relational and interactional approach. Relevant to this argument, Bergmeier et al. (2016) observed mothers and children just before and during mealtime. They found that mothers' responsiveness to their children's perspective and needs increased from the time when food was being prepared to when it was being eaten. As well, a mother's level of responsiveness was negatively related to her child's fussy eating. Thus mothers appeared to be setting up a situation in which compliance would be more likely, rather than becoming entangled in negative actions and affect.

Another setting that involves parent–child interaction in the reciprocity domain focuses on parents' use of technology. McDaniel and Radesky (2018), for example, asked mothers to rate how much difficulty they had resisting the use of technical devices. Mothers who said they could not resist checking new messages on their cell phones when they were alerted to their existence, who often thought about calls or messages they might receive on their phones, and who felt that they used their phones too much also reported more technology-based interruptions of their interactions with their preschoolers. Their preschoolers, in turn, were more likely to exhibit both internalizing and externalizing problems. Interestingly, the same relation did not hold for fathers. Studies assessing direction of effect in the context of "technoference" are needed.

## ■ CONCLUSION

The reciprocity domain is a happy one, with parent and child engaged in a mutually harmonious and egalitarian relationship. Goals are shared, and cooperation comes naturally rather than being forced. Threats of punishment and hope of reward do not have a role to play in this domain. Indeed, the introduction of reward for compliance may well neutralize or even undermine the effects of responsiveness to the child's requests (see Chapter 5). Reciprocity between parent and child, along with interactions in the protection domain, form the two bases or foundations of effective parenting, so that the learning of values is facilitated in the other three domains.

It is important to note that not all children's requests need to be accommodated in the reciprocity domain. Requests should be reasonable ones, not only in kind, but in number. Perhaps one guideline for what is reasonable with respect to number of requests has to do with the extent to which children are compliant. If they are difficult and uncooperative, it could be that parent compliance needs to be augmented; that is, more resources need to be put into the socialization bank.

In this chapter, I have suggested that different kinds of mutuality in interactions may serve somewhat different functions. Efforts made to accommodate children's requests are investments in future interactions, so that favors are more likely to be returned. Synchronous interactions—where both members of the dyad participate in taking turns, and where the interaction is accompanied by positive emotions—may be important for developing social skills, including cooperative and positive interactions with others. Both of these forms of interaction are central for successful socialization.

## ■ A POSTSCRIPT

When children are distressed, it is not difficult to offer some form of comfort or aid. In contrast, when children who are in a positive frame of mind want to engage in some activity that requires the parent to be a partner, acquiescence may not be quite so compelling, as Andrew Solomon observed in a review of Jennifer Senior's book *All Joy and No Fun:*

> Over and over again I find myself bored by what I'm doing with my children: How many times can we read "Angelina Ballerina" or watch a "Bob the Builder" video? And yet I remind myself that such intimate shared moments, snuggling close, provide the ultimate meaning of life. . . . If I lost all my emails I'd manage, and if I lost my children, I'd never recover; yet still I sometimes find it hard to stay in the moment with them. (*www.nytimes.com/2014/02/02/books/review/all-joy-and-no-fun-by-jennifer-senior.html*)

**CHAPTER 1 SCENARIOS REVISITED**

I return again to the sample scenarios from Chapter 1, this time in the reciprocity domain. They are reproduced in Box 4.1, along with possible parenting reactions.

In the first case, where Alan asks if he and his mother can watch planes taking off, his mother in both Alternatives A and C misses an opportunity to put money into the socialization bank. In Alternative B, Alan's mother complies with her son's reasonable request, and so increases the probability that her son will comply with her wish at some future point in time. She may, for example, find that he is more likely, once they are on the plane, to comply with her request that he not kick the seat of the passenger sitting in front of him.

In the second scenario, a father agrees to play with his daughter, but tries to direct the interaction (Alternative B)—not the best approach. In Alternative A, he fully complies with her reasonable request. Alternative C, of course, represents a missed opportunity for facilitating future compliance.

---

**BOX 4.1.** Scenarios from the Reciprocity Domain

*Alan (5 years old) and his mother are waiting in the airport terminal for their boarding call. Mother is texting, and Alan is bored. He asks his mother if they can go and watch some planes taking off.*

A. Mother says they can't, because they might miss the boarding announcement.

B. Mother says they can, if they don't go too far so they miss the boarding announcement.

C. Mother tells Alan to sit quietly, and she continues texting.

*Stella (8 years old) asks her father, who is watching the news, to play a card game with her. Dad finds this particular card game especially boring.*

A. Dad says, "OK, let's play for a while."

B. Dad says, "Why don't we play a different card game?"

C. Dad says, "Not right now, Stella. I'm watching the news."

**CHAPTER 5**

# Learning Values in the Control Domain

*Discipline and Reward*

In the protection domain, children learn to trust their caregivers and thus to believe that the caregivers' requests for compliance are in their best interests. In the reciprocity domain, children come to comply happily and easily with requests for compliance, because they and their caregivers are caught up in a mutually responsive and warm relationship. These two domains form the basis or foundation of a positive and amicable parent–child relationship—a foundation that makes it easier for parents subsequently to encourage their children's adoption of specific values and associated thoughts and actions. Because they trust their parents to be wiser, and because they are part of an exchange relationship, children are more open to accepting or adopting the values their parents are promoting. In this chapter and the next two—the chapters on control, guided learning, and group participation—I turn to a discussion of exactly how this adoption is achieved.

The acquisition of values in the control domain involves the use of discipline and reward to promote positive behavior and discourage negative behavior. In the guided learning domain, children are taught what is appropriate behavior and what is not; in the group participation domain, they learn from models and from engaging with others in socially appropriate actions. In planning this book, I spent some time thinking about the order in which these three topics should

82

be discussed. By starting with the control domain, I might leave the impression that this is the most important or most effective way of promoting acceptable thinking and acting. But that is not necessarily the case. In the end I have decided to deal with the control domain first, simply because it is the area of socialization that has received the most research attention, and also because discipline is an area of particularly great concern to most parents.

From an evolutionary perspective, control is important in order to achieve social harmony and avoid harmful dissension (Boehm, 2000). To be able to function effectively in the group, its members must obey and accept cultural rules, even when this means that personal desires have to be inhibited. Accordingly, the control domain involves conflict, with younger group members wanting one thing and older, more experienced, members requiring something different. This is how the control domain differs from the reciprocity domain, where compliance is willingly given, and where there is no conflict because goals are shared. In the control domain, parents take advantage of the fact that they possess more resources they can use to alter their children's undesirable behavior and to encourage their children's desirable behavior. In this way, they train them to become successful and accepted members of the social community, thereby promoting their potential for mating and reproductive success.

All this, by the way, is not to suggest that children are lacking in their own resources and ability to influence their parents' behavior, as noted in Chapter 1. But parents do have greater control over material resources, as well as greater physical size and strength. Additionally, their superior knowledge and experience enables them to persuade effectively through reasoning and explanation, which are also part of the control domain.

There are significant challenges in the control domain. The first is that values be internalized. It is too demanding for parents or other members of the social community to keep its members under constant surveillance. The only way that socialization can succeed in this domain is if a child being socialized takes over the job of surveillance by developing a self-guiding conscience. Another challenge is that interactions in the control domain are often heated, with both members in the exchange angry, frustrated, or disappointed. These strong negative emotions make constructive interaction somewhat more difficult than it is in the guided learning or group participation domain.

## ■ THE CONTROL DOMAIN AND VALUE LEARNING

What kinds of experiences do children have in the control domain, and how does that affect their learning of values? Following are a few examples of narratives (reproduced as written) that were collected in my lab and that involve undergraduate students' recollections of a time when they learned an important value in the control domain (Vinik et al., 2013; Vinik, 2013). Whereas the narratives may not be totally accurate depictions of past events, they do reflect perceptions and memories of events that provided the material for acquiring a particular belief or value.

The narratives our students provided were not all in the control domain. There were, however, more narratives in that domain than in any of the other domains. Moreover, many more of them involved responses to children's misbehavior than responses to their positive behavior.

Note in these narratives the many different kinds of antisocial actions, as well as the many different kinds of strategies parents employed in their responses. The former included lack of self-control (eating too much dessert), being mean to a sibling, stealing from a classmate, ignoring an admonition to be careful not to hurt oneself, lying to a teacher, playing with fire, and not assuming responsibility for one's obligations. Parents' strategies, in turn, included criticism; criticism and explanation; expressions of anger and withdrawal of privileges; a reminder that parental advice should be heeded after the failure to do so led to personal harm; lecture and punishment; explanation, along with acknowledgment of the child's wishes and compromise; and decreased nagging and more subtle reminders with increasing age. In the remainder of this chapter, these and other parenting strategies are discussed in terms of their relative effectiveness in teaching values and acceptable behavior.

### The Narratives

At the end of each narrative, information about the student's sex and ethnicity is provided, along with the student's age at the time of the event he or she was describing.

"i learned not to be a glutton from my family. i used to really like eating dessert, always extra dessert and someone on my Mom's side at a family thing made a crack about all my dessert eating and so did someone on my Dad's side, so i felt bad for eating so much cake. i also realized why they were all concerned, for my health and heart it was unhealthy for me to be eating so much dessert and i learned another important lesson in self control." (Female, age 13, Western European)

"I remembered that my brother did something wrong (which I could have misjudged), and I felt so ashamed and angry about it because he did it in front of my whole family. I slapped him. . . . Also, when I was small, I used to tease/ scold my brother for his uncompetitiveness or things he did wrong. Often it would develop into a quarrel or fight. . . . After all these events, my parents would lecture me again and again and again and again . . . on brothers should love and take care each other, not quarreling all the time." (Male, age 10, East Asian)

"This event occurred when I was in kindergarten. It was snack time; me and my two friends ate our snacks. We then spotted a classmate's snack, full of cookies, left alone on his desk; he had gone to the washroom. Me and my two friends stole some of the cookies; however, we got caught by our classmate. He went and told the teacher, who got mad immediately. She gave us a big lecture, asked us to apologize to the classmate, and called home to let our parents know about our behavior. At that moment, all I wanted to do was punch my classmate in the face; I even gave him the 'buddy, you're dead after school' look. Later that day when my mom came to pick me up, my teacher had a long discussion with her. My mom got mad and I ended up being grounded for one week. During that week, I realized the trouble I got into and the fun I had to stay away from for stealing a cookie. From then on, I never stole ever again." (Female, age 4, South Asian)

"This was due to an accident which I had while playing with my cousin. It was at my maternal grandmother's house and we were running around playing catch. My mother had told me countless times whenever I ran past her to stop running in case I fell. But I did not heed her advice and continued until I hit my forehead on the corner of the door and had to be rushed to the hospital for stitches. The ride to the hospital was a little blur as all I knew was my head being covered by a towel and my mum frantically driving me there. I was so afraid and wished that I had never ignored her warning. My mother then told me after the stitches that I should be more obedient and she would never had stopped me from playing if she knew it was safe. It really taught me to listen when parents give their advice." (Female, age 6, East Asian)

"In elementary school I was in deep trouble for lying to the teacher. When the principal and teacher told my father, he was very disappointed. In order to set me straight, my father lectured me and punished me. I still remember the lecture he gave as he had a very negative tone. I then learned to be as honest as I can be, because trust is key in developing relationships with people. This event has stuck with me for all my life and I try my best to be honest to my peers." (Male, age 9, South Asian)

"It is probably accurate to say that most children, especially boys, are fascinated by fire at some point in their childhood. This fascination can be observed when the child plays with matches or burns leaves with a magnifying glass. I happened to do both of these things. One day, my father caught my playing with matches. He didn't scold me, which I found to be very 'cool' at the time, and I suppose was a factor in my taking his advice to heart. He simply warned me about a friend of his who was burned badly when they were kids. He stressed how important it is to be safe around fire. Of course he didn't deny the fun in playing with it. So he offered me a compromise: If I would stop playing with the matches, etc. he would let me help with fireworks the next time we did them (In a safe manner of course). I decided that if he was warning me about this there would be legitimate reason to listen, and so I did." (Male, age 8, Western European)

"My mom used to help me with my homework a lot, with budgeting my time, getting things done, and going to bed at a reasonable hour. However, around grade 11 she taught me how to be responsible for myself. She began to nag me a lot less about homework, practicing piano, etc. and since I was older and would often stay up later, instead of insisting I go to bed she would just go to her room around 10:00–10:30 and say 'I'm going to bed'. From this I began to learn to self-discipline myself; since no one was telling me to stop what I was doing and go to bed, for a while I stayed up way too late doing point-less things but gradually I became more responsible and now am able to tell myself that even though I might want to stay up later, I should go to bed so I will have energy the next day." (Female, age 16, Western European)

## ■ TWO APPROACHES TO CONTROL

Views on control have emerged from two quite different directions. One has to do with forms of discipline and how they affect the learning of values. The second has to do with styles of parenting and their relation not only to value learning, but to other aspects of socioemotional development. I discuss each in turn.

### Forms of Discipline and Internalization of Values

*Psychoanalytic Theory*

The first formal analysis of discipline and internalization of values came from Sigmund Freud (1930). Freud argued that whenever parents impose demands on their children, feelings of hostility and resentment are inevitable results. (In modern terminology, this would be called "reactance," or the desire to do the opposite of what is asked.) Children do not express their hostility, however, because they are afraid their parents will stop loving them or will even abandon them. And so the hostility is repressed. This repression is maintained when children adopt their parents' rules and prohibitions in an attempt to gain parental approval or love, as well as when they internalize or take over the parental role. Punishment for transgression, one of the features of parenting behavior that is internalized (or introjected), is transformed into self-punishment or guilt after deviation—that is, into an emotion that resembles anxiety about parental punishment and fear of abandonment. In this way, guilt avoidance underlies internalization of societal standards and leads to actions that accord with those standards even in the absence of external surveillance. Freud's analysis, as well as emphasizing fear of loss of love as a primary motivator of socially acceptable behavior, also provided the basis for the notion that a parent's values are taken over with no modification (i.e., that values are transmitted rather than constructed by a child).

## Social Learning Theory

Freud's ideas offered a rich way of conceptualizing human development, but they were difficult to evaluate scientifically. Indeed, Freud's followers argued that Freudian hypotheses were not amenable to scientific testing, but could be assessed only through use of the psychoanalytic method—that is, the free associations of patients undergoing analysis or the behavior of children during structured play. However, beginning in the late 1930s and continuing into the early 1960s, academic psychologists who were interested in developing a theory of personality, and who were impressed by Freud's many insights, found a way to wed his theory with a more scientific approach. The scientific approach was that of Hullian stimulus–response theory (e.g., Dollard, Doob, Miller, Mowrer, & Sears, 1939; Sears, Whiting, Nowlis, & Sears, 1953). The combination of Freudian ideas and stimulus–response theory was labeled "social learning theory" and guided a great deal of developmental theorizing for a considerable period of time.

Particularly important for the study of the internalization of values or conscience was *Patterns of Child Rearing* by Sears, Maccoby, and Levin (1957). The book was a summary of findings based on interviews of 379 mothers about their childrearing practices. Sears et al. focused on topics that played a central role in Freudian theory—aggression, dependency, discipline, and sex roles—and attempted to apply learning theory concepts to understand their development. In the case of discipline or control strategies, Sears et al. found that mothers' reports of how they disciplined their children for misbehavior could be placed into two categories: "love-oriented" and "object-oriented." The former included praise, social isolation, withdrawal of affection and reasoning, and the latter tangible rewards, deprivation of material objects or privileges, and physical punishment. The approach that worked best for the development of conscience or internalization of values was withdrawal of love from a mother who was warm. The explanation provided was that losing the mother's attention motivates the child to take on characteristics of the mother, and that the characteristics most likely to be taken on are those associated with the love withdrawal. The warmer or more reinforcing the parent, the greater the desire to become like the parent. In the case of object-oriented discipline, the only motivation is to avoid punishment and to hide from the parent.

## Martin Hoffman's Analysis of Parental Discipline

An influential chapter by Martin Hoffman (1970b) in *Carmichael's Manual of Child Psychology* set out a new direction for the study of socialization processes. In a review and expansion of existing research and theory with respect to discipline and value internalization, Hoffman made a more fine-grained differentiation among forms of discipline than had Sears and his colleagues. Rather than talking about object-oriented punishment and withdrawal of love and reasoning as control techniques, he distinguished three approaches to control: "power assertion," "love withdrawal," and "induction." Power assertion includes physical punishment, deprivation of material objects or privileges, application of force, or threat of any of these. Love withdrawal refers to direct, but not physical expression of, disapproval. And induction is the provision of explanations and appeals to the child's pride and desire to be mature. In the induction category, Hoffman singled out one particular parenting strategy that he labeled "other-oriented"—an approach that involves making children aware of the consequences of their misdeeds for others. Hoffman also distinguished four aspects of internalization or moral development: resistance to temptation, guilt after deviation, moral judgment depicting an internal as opposed to external orientation, and confession and acceptance of responsibility for a given antisocial act. In his survey of the research literature, he found that on average, power assertion was negatively related to internalization, induction was positively related, and there was no relation with withdrawal of love. He also noted that parental warmth alone was positively related to internalization. Although there were fewer studies with fathers, those that existed did not show the same pattern of effectiveness; rather, all seemed to be equivalent in their impact.

Hoffman offered a series of explanations for his observations. He suggested that power–assertive techniques anger the child because they both challenge the child's autonomy and also provide an antisocial model for handling anger. Power assertion, in contrast to other-oriented discipline, also focuses the child's attention on the self rather than the harmed object, and so its use does not take advantage of the child's empathic capacity. Finally, when children are in a high state of arousal, their ability to utilize cues in the surrounding situation is limited. Although most of these negative features of power assertion are less likely to be present in the case of withdrawal of love, this latter strategy still does not focus the child on harm done to others.

Although Hoffman emphasized the importance of induction or reasoning, he did not suggest that either power assertion or withdrawal of love is a technique that should be avoided entirely (Hoffman, 1982). A moderate level of power assertion or disapproval, he maintained, is necessary in order to gain the child's attention and ensure that the information contained in the parent's reasoning is listened to and assimilated.

## Attributional Analyses

Attribution theorists maintained, along with Hoffman, that punishment has a role to play in the discipline process, but that the level of punishment must be an optimal one. By "optimal," they meant that it should be just sufficient, and no more, to obtain compliance. Lepper (1983), for example, noted that children who are mildly punished for playing with particular toys, as opposed to severely punished, are more likely to refrain from playing with those toys at a later time when they are not under surveillance (Freedman, 1965). Calling on the "minimal sufficiency principle," Lepper suggested that in the case of severe punishment, children can easily attribute their positive behavior to external demands. As a result, they continue to behave in an antisocial way when those external pressures are not in evidence. When punishment is just sufficient to promote compliance, however, it becomes more difficult to attribute compliance to a fear of external consequences; thus compliance is seen as internally motivated and therefore appropriate, regardless of external contingencies.

## A Reconceptualization of the Relative Effectiveness of Reasoning and Power Assertion

Although it was generally maintained by developmentalists that reasoning is a more effective approach to modifying children's antisocial behavior than power assertion or punishment, Grusec and Goodnow (1994), taking a social cognitive approach, pointed out many instances in the research literature where this was not the case. Outcomes depended on a number of variables, including children's age, sex, and temperament, as well as the nature of the misdeed under consideration, whether the socializing agent was a mother or a father, and the cultural context. Additionally, they noted that a wide variety of discipline strategies were lumped together within the two categories of reasoning and power assertion, with no attempt to differentiate among them in terms of their effectiveness. Other-oriented induction, statements of norms, statements of practical consequences, and explanations seen by a child as unconvincing do not produce the same results. Nor do physical punishment, social isolation, withdrawal of privileges, disapproval, and humiliation. Grusec and Goodnow also noted that parents use different techniques, depending on the nature of the particular misdeed to which they are responding (Grusec & Kuczynski, 1980), as well as that abusive or harsh parents are more likely to use the same approach, regardless of the nature of the misdeed (Trickett & Kuczynski, 1986).

In light of these various observations, Grusec and Goodnow (1994) suggested that socialization of positive social behavior should be seen as the result of two events: the child's accurate perception of the parent's value, and the child's willingness to accept and act in accord with that value. Thus a child may know what the parent's value is, but may not be willing to comply with it. Or a child may be quite willing to comply, but may not perceive the value correctly. In both these cases, then, there will be no internalization of that value. Only when perception is accurate and willingness to comply is high will the outcome be a positive one.

### ACCURATE PERCEPTION

Accurate perception is facilitated by a number of events, including clear, frequent, and consistent expression of messages. It also requires that messages be matched to the child's level of cognitive development, such as the ability to take the perspective of another person or to understand complex rationales. Moderate levels of power assertion force attention to and underline the importance of the message. Implicit messages (e.g., "This is a house, not a stable") force attention because they require decoding. Variables involved in accurate perception are listed in Table 5.1.

ACCEPTANCE

Acceptance is made up of three variables: the child's perception of the appropriateness of a request, the child's motivation, and the child's perception that a value is self-generated. The first variable, appropriateness, includes beliefs that the parent is making a fair and reasonable request, that the request makes sense, and that the request is in keeping with the values of the particular cultural context in which the child is operating. Strict parenting, for example, is more normative and considered more

| TABLE 5.1. Features of Accurate Perception and Acceptance |
| --- |
| *Accurate perception of message* |
| • Message is clear, redundant, and consistent, and is fitted to existing schemas (understandable, relevant, and not tangential).<br>• Child's attention is captured.<br>• Message requires decoding, which prompts comprehension.<br>• Importance to parent and parent's positive intention are conveyed. |
| *Acceptance of message* |
| *Perceived as appropriate*<br>• Message is fitted to nature of misdeed, has truth/value; due process is observed; and expected procedures are followed.<br>• Message is seen as well intentioned.<br>• Message is fitted to child's temperament, mood, and developmental status. |
| *Motivating*<br>• Empathy is aroused.<br>• Importance to parent is stressed.<br>• Desire to identify with parent is promoted.<br>• Autonomy is supported.<br>• Indirect and implicit messages are accompanied by humor. |
| *Felt as self-generated*<br>• Threats to autonomy are minimized.<br>• Decoding is required.<br>• Child's discounting patterns are taken into account. |

acceptable in some cultures than it is in others. The second variable, motivation for compliance, can involve threats to feelings of security, levels of empathic arousal, the extent to which compliance is seen to be important to the parent, the degree to which the relationship encourages reciprocity, and the desire to please a warm and loving parent. The third variable, perception of self-generation, can occur either when autonomy support is high or when the message needs decoding (e.g., "Who was your servant last year?") Variables involved in acceptance are also listed in Table 5.1.

## EVIDENCE

Various aspects of the Grusec and Goodnow (1994) model have been tested. Knafo and Schwartz (2003), for example, measured accuracy by correlating parents' reports of values they wished to instill in their children and the children's report of the values they thought their parents wanted them to have. They found that accuracy was associated with a number of variables, including the extent to which parents agreed on the values they held, as well as parents' warmth and their use of reasoning. Accuracy was negatively correlated with autocratic parenting and with indifferent parenting. In another study, acceptance was associated with a close parent–child relationship and with consideration for the child's autonomy (Barni, Ranieri, Scabini, & Rosnati, 2011). In keeping with the argument that accurate perception and acceptance are both required for the display of positive social behavior, Padilla-Walker (2007) found that accurate perception of maternal values was related to adolescent values, but only when acceptance was high, and not when it was low. In a study of mother–adolescent dyads (Gath & Grusec, 2018), it was observed that mothers' moral identity (presumably a reflection of the extent to which she offered clear messages about positive social behavior) predicted adolescents' generosity and moral reasoning, but only when the mothers were warm and involved with their children.

## SUMMARY ■ ■ ■ ■ ■ ■ ■ ■ ■ ■ ■ ■ ■ ■ ■ ■ ■ ■ ■ ■ ■ ■ ■ ■ ■ ■ ■ ■ ■ ■ ■ ■ ■ ■

The formal study of discipline and value internalization has a long history in psychology, beginning with Freud. Freud introduced the notions of love withdrawal, self-punishment or guilt, and conscience or internalization of societal standards. Subsequently, social learning theorists compared two forms of discipline—love-oriented (which included reasoning) and object-oriented—and concluded that withdrawal of love from a warm mother is the most effective approach to discipline. A major step forward came with Hoffman's emphasis on induction or reasoning, and particularly on what he labeled "other-oriented" induction, or concern for the impact of one's actions on others. Hoffman suggested that this approach to discipline is superior because it takes advantage of the child's empathic capacities. However, neither Hoffman nor attribution theorists denied the important role of power assertion in effective discipline. Mild levels of punishment catch the child's attention, so that the information parents are presenting is assimilated. Also, compliance after punishment that is just sufficient can be attributed to internal factors, whereas punishment that is too severe allows positive behavior to be attributed to external pressure; when that pressure is no longer in evidence, positive behavior declines. Finally, the Grusec and Goodnow model described the complexity of discipline, noting multiple forms of reasoning and power assertion as well as interactions between these forms, features of children, nature of the misdeed, and so on. They suggested that socialization in the control domain be considered as a function of children's accurate perception and acceptance of the parent's message. With only one of these outcomes, the child is left to accept a value the parent did not intend to teach, or to reject a value the parent clearly held.

## Parenting Style

I turn now to the second major research approach to socialization and discipline—"parenting style." Parenting styles are reflections of attitudes toward a child that create an emotional climate in which value learning takes place. They comprise variables such as punitiveness, strictness, warmth, and rejection. Sometimes they are translated into two orthogonal dimensions, such as warmth versus hostility and autonomy support versus control (with control having a completely negative connotation) (Baldwin, 1955).

### Kurt Lewin and Alfred Baldwin

Work on parenting styles had its origins in social psychology and the research of Kurt Lewin on group atmosphere (Maccoby, 1992, 2015). Distressed by the growth of totalitarianism and anti-Semitism in Europe just prior to World War II, Lewin and his colleagues wanted to find out how people respond to autocratic direction (Lewin, Lippitt, &

White, 1939). And so they undertook a series of experiments intended to mimic different political ideologies. With young boys as research participants, they ran recreational and crafts groups in three different ways. In the first ("democratic"), members were encouraged to make decisions themselves, with a rational and dispassionate leader encouraging decision making, offering suggestions if requested, and providing feedback on the group's functioning. In the second group ("authoritarian"), the leaders, who were aloof, decided what the group would do and who would do it, as well as offering praise or blame without giving clear reasons for what the boys had done to deserve it. In the third group ("laissez-faire"), friendly leaders explained what materials were available, but did nothing else. The democratic group, not unexpectedly, did best, with its members cooperating with the leader and working well in the leader's absence. Boys in the authoritarian group, in spite of privately expressing dislike for the leader, competed for attention and praise. When they were left alone, however, they stopped working and engaged in wild horseplay (possibly an expression of suppressed tension). Finally, the laissez-faire group was disorganized and ineffective in its work.

Alfred Baldwin was a graduate student at Harvard when Lewin was a visiting faculty member there, and he soon recognized the importance of Lewin's work for understanding family functioning. When Baldwin set up his own research program, he translated Lewin's groups into parenting styles (Baldwin, 1955). However, he distinguished between "scientific" democracy and "warm" democracy, with the former involving emotional detachment, and the latter affection and empathy for the child's point of view. He found that warm democratic parenting, which gave the child a great deal of freedom, was associated with stronger intellectual development, more spontaneity, and less anxiety than the other parenting styles. However, it was also a predictor of increased antisocial behavior.

### Diana Baumrind

The analysis of parenting styles by Baldwin underlined the harmful outcomes of authoritarian childrearing practices as well as the importance of parental warmth. Parents should not be focused simply on gaining their children's obedience and deference, and they should express unconditional acceptance and love toward their children. This conclusion was seen by many as a recommendation for unconditional permissiveness—a position with which Diana Baumrind strongly disagreed (Maccoby, 2015). Baumrind (1971) emphasized the importance of setting standards of behavior for children and distinguished between two forms of control, one positive and the other negative.

Baumrind's categories of parenting styles are well known. The "authoritative" style began with Baldwin's democratic style but was expanded to include the imposition of high standards and demands for mature behavior, as well as reasoning, negotiating, taking the child's point of view into account, and encouraging autonomy. The "authoritarian" style was characterized by high demandingness and low responsiveness, with authoritarian parents being rigid, harsh, and strict. The "permissive" style was exhibited by parents who were overly responsive to children's demands and inconsistent with respect to enforcement of rules. It was the authoritative style that Baumrind found to be associated with social responsibility, peer competence, cooperation with adults, social dominance, nonconformity, and purposiveness.

In a relatively recent elaboration of her position, Baumrind (2012) wrote further about parenting styles and their relation to discipline. For Baumrind, power assertion and control are interchangeable; power assertion means, in the disciplinary context, force applied by parents in a conflict of wills with their children. What matters is the way the force is applied. In "confrontive" control (the authoritative parenting style), power assertion is accompanied by responsiveness to the child's wishes and needs, as well as the use of explanations. In "coercive" control (the authoritarian style), control encompasses force, unambivalent exercise of power, and discouragement of defiance. Because confrontive power assertion is overt, direct, rational, and goal-directed, it leaves room for the child to choose among complying, arguing, seeking a mutually acceptable compromise, or paying a known price for noncompliance. When there is disagreement between parent and child, then, the child uses these constructive techniques, whereas in the case of coercive control, the child's reaction is more likely to be evasion or subversion, along with resentment, conflict, and withdrawal. Authoritative parents balance demands for conformity in accord with legitimate social constraints and allowing their children to make choices. By allowing children to choose how they wish to deal with parental demands, parents offset any negative effects that control might have on the children's sense of self-efficacy and intrinsic motivation. In this analysis, Baumrind emphasizes that reasoning on its own is not sufficient for successful socialization and that some pressure is required. In this observation, of course, she reflects the similar position set forth by Hoffman (1982). Hoffman suggests that some degree of power assertion is necessary to gain children's attention so they can hear their parents' messages. Baumrind suggests that some degree of power assertion is necessary to ensure that children understand the choices they are being asked to make.

## Distinguishing Parenting Practices from Their Context

The concept of parenting styles was elaborated in a paper by Darling and Steinberg (1993), who began with the observation that authoritative and authoritarian parenting do not have the same outcomes in all cultures. For example, authoritative parenting is associated with academic achievement for European American adolescents but not for Asian American or African American adolescents, and authoritarian parenting with timid and anxious behavior for European American children but with assertive behavior for African American girls. Darling and Steinberg proposed that these sorts of apparently contradictory findings necessitate the drawing of a distinction between the substance of parenting practices and the context in which they occur. The former involves such strategies as spanking, showing an interest in children's activities, and requiring children to do their homework, whereas the latter involves the emotional climate expressed by parental behaviors such as tone of voice, body language, inattention, and bursts of temper. Style conveys how the parent feels about the child, while content conveys how the parent feels about the child's behavior. This approach, in some respects at least, maps onto the Grusec and Goodnow (1994) analysis in terms of accurate perception and acceptance, with practices linked to accurate perception and style to acceptance.

## Behavioral and Psychological Control

In addition to authoritative and authoritarian control, researchers have identified two other forms of control: "behavioral" and "psychological" (Barber, 1996). Behavioral control refers to reasonable setting of rules for children's behavior and reasonable enforcement of those rules. When it is unreasonable or occurs at too high a level, it predicts maladjustment. When it is too low, it is associated with externalizing problems, including antisocial behavior, truancy, and drug use (Barber & Harmon, 2002; Crouter & Head, 2002). In other words, it is autonomy-supportive in the sense of requiring only a moderate level of pressure for the achievement of compliance.

Psychological control refers to attempts to influence a child's emotional state in an effort to gain obedience; it includes guilt induction, withdrawal of love, and intrusiveness. Psychologically controlling parents are manipulative and insensitive to their children's emotional needs—a feature of parenting that undermines the children's self-esteem and self-identity. Psychological control is associated with internalizing problems, such as anxiety, depression, loneliness, low academic achievement, low self-esteem, low self-reliance, and self-derogation (Barber & Harmon, 2002). In a meta-analysis, Kuppens, Laurent, Heyvaert, and Onghena (2013) also found some evidence that psychological control was related to children's relational aggression— that is, behavior intended to damage another person's self-esteem or social status. The link is not surprising, given that children learn from their experience with psychological control that the manipulation of a social relationship is an effective way of achieving personal goals. Thus a child who threatens to end a friendship as a way of manipulating or modifying a peer's behavior is similar to a parent who threatens to withdraw love as a way of manipulating or modifying a child's behavior. Kuppens et al. also found that the relation between psychological control and relational aggression was moderated by age, with stronger effects occurring during adolescence. Presumably this age effect reflects adolescents' increasing concern with self-esteem and self-identity.

## The Self-Determination Perspective

Another way to understand control and its different manifestations is from the perspective of self-determination theory (Deci & Ryan, 1985; Grolnick et al., 1997). According to self-determination theory (which I have introduced in my discussion of internalization in Chapter 1), although children find many activities intrinsically rewarding, there are other behaviors that are not intrinsically rewarding and that must be encouraged for internalization to take place. Internalization is facilitated by autonomy support in the form of gentle control and the provision of appropriate choice; the setting of clear expectations (structure); the provision of explanation; and interpersonal involvement manifested by warmth, caring, and a demonstration of interest in the child. Autonomy support aids the perception that behavior is self-generated rather than externally imposed. Structure enables children to know what is appropriate action. Explanation helps them understand why an action has personal utility. And interpersonal involvement makes children willing to accept the structure.

Autonomy support is undermined if support is intrusive (e.g., helping with or checking children's homework when it has not been requested), even though such parenting action does communicate caring. Intrusive support has particularly negative consequences, at least in the area of school achievement, for children who are less academically successful—presumably because they are more sensitive to the inference of incompetence that such parenting offers (Ng, Kenney-Benson, & Pomerantz, 2004).

## SUMMARY ■ ■ ■ ■ ■ ■ ■ ■ ■ ■ ■ ■ ■ ■ ■ ■ ■ ■ ■ ■ ■ ■ ■ ■ ■ ■ ■ ■ ■ ■ ■ ■ ■ ■ ■ ■ ■ ■

For more than half a century, parenting styles, like discipline practices, have played a major role in understanding socialization. Research on these styles has focused in particular on forms of control. Thus the question has been not *whether* control should be exercised, but *how* it should be exercised (Maccoby, 2015). The answer seems to be that it should be confrontive, not coercive. It should include reasonable limits on the child's behavior. It should be applied in an autonomy-supportive way that includes taking the child's perspective, giving the child choices, and reasoning. Finally, control should be accompanied by structure (a clear setting out of rules) and by warmth.

There is certainly nothing in this position that contradicts the idea of discipline as a combination of reasoning and reasonable amounts of power assertion, and as the result of an interaction between accurate perception of rules of behavior (structure) and acceptance of those rules. In the final analysis, the two approaches complement each other quite nicely. Given that they both address how antisocial behavior is modified, this is as it should be.

## ■ MODERATORS OF DISCIPLINE EFFECTIVENESS, AND DIFFERENT FORMS OF REASONING AND POWER ASSERTION COMPARED

### Moderators of Discipline Effectiveness

The effects of discipline are moderated by a considerable array of variables. A sample of these moderators includes a child's temperament, age, and sex; the sex of the parent; and the affective and cultural context in which the discipline is administered.

### Child's Temperament

Research that addresses temperament as a moderating influence in the socialization process is most frequently guided by a transactional/ dual-risk model. According to this model, problematic parenting is more likely to have a negative impact on children with difficult temperaments than on children with easy temperaments. Children who are fearful or timid, for example, exhibit high levels of externalizing behavior and low levels of positive behavior when they are harshly parented, whereas fearless children seem not to be negatively affected by such parenting (Kochanska, 1995; Kochanska, Aksan, & Joy, 2007; Lengua, 2008).

It is not always fearful or timid children who are especially affected by certain forms of problem parenting. Cornell and Frick (2007), for example, found with young children that maternal inconsistent discipline (although not authoritarian parenting) predicted low levels of empathy—an important component of prosocial behavior—but only for *fearless* and not for fearful ones. In a longitudinal study, Chaparro and Grusec (2016) found the same relation for adolescents whose mothers (but not their fathers) were inconsistent disciplinarians (but not authoritarian). Chaparro and Grusec suggested that fearful or neurotic adolescents are more wary of possible punishment, and so they are more likely to comply with parental directives even when those directives are inconsistently enforced. Fearless adolescents are less cautious and therefore more willing to take a chance that they might be able to avoid punishment for noncompliance. One implication of these findings with respect to temperament could be that it is important to discipline fearful children gently and fearless children consistently.

### Child's Age

Links between harsh parenting and externalizing behavior are stronger for older children than for younger ones, perhaps because older children are more likely to see such parenting as infringing on their sense of autonomy (Rothbaum & Weisz, 1994). Young children also evaluate physical punishment by mothers more favorably than do older children (Siegal & Cowen, 1984). In a study of Canadian and Chinese children, Helwig, To, Wang, Liu, and Yang (2014) found that both cultural groups evaluated reasoning more favorably than either withdrawal of love or shaming at all ages, but that withdrawal of love and shaming were increasingly negatively valued with age.

Presumably children, as they age, develop an increasing appreciation for the importance of long-term goals that are fostered by reasoning, rather than short-term goals such as immediate compliance that are fostered by different forms of punishment. They also develop greater sophistication with respect to possible negative outcomes of discipline techniques. The content of reasoning is also important with respect to age; rationales need to match the level of the child's comprehension. And young children are less able to appreciate subtle methods of delivery, such as messages spoken in a "kidding" fashion, a sarcastic way, or a neutral tone of voice (Bugental, Kaswan, Love, & Fox, 1970; Morton & Trehub, 2001).

In addition to changing reactions to and evaluations of discipline techniques, children also change with age in their views of the kinds of behavior parents have a right to control. Thus older children see many more issues as being under their own jurisdiction and therefore not subject to parental dictates (Smetana, Robinson, & Rote, 2015). The decreasing effectiveness of discipline in general, as children grow older, was highlighted in a longitudinal study by Kerr, Stattin, and Özdemir (2012). They asked about the direction of effect between parenting styles and adolescent adjustment (school problems, externalizing problems, delinquency, loitering on the streets, intoxication frequency, low self-esteem, and depressed mood) in adolescents who were first assessed when they were 13 and 14 years old and then again 2 years later. They found that adolescent adjustment was a stronger and more robust predictor of parenting style than vice versa at the second time point, suggesting that the impact of parent discipline may wane with age. The finding by Kerr et al. does highlight the fact that other strategies—monitoring and disclosure, which I discuss below—need to come into greater play as children age.

### Sex of Child

Maternal caregiving is linked more strongly to externalizing behavior for preadolescent boys than it is for girls (Rothbaum & Weisz, 1994). Boys are more likely than girls to be involved in coercive cycles of escalating negative behavior with their mothers (Patterson, 1980). Mothers who endorsed demands for family deference and parental respect at birth had children who at 12 years of age displayed externalizing problems, but this relation held only for boys and not for girls (Awong, Grusec, & Sorenson, 2005). These are examples of studies suggesting that boys are more easily involved in negative exchanges than girls, at least with their mothers.

### Sex of Parent

Mothers and fathers have different disciplinary styles, which leads children to evaluate their parents differently for the same action. This different evaluation, in turn, has an impact on how children respond to the same form of discipline (Grusec & Goodnow, 1994). Fathers are more likely to want simply to end a conflict, whereas mothers want the conflict to be settled in an amicable fashion (Vuchinich, Emery, & Cassidy, 1988). And children believe that fathers not only would, but in fact should, use more power-assertive techniques than mothers (Dadds, Sheffield, & Holbeck, 1990; Siegal & Barclay, 1985).

### Affective Context

The emotional context in which power assertion and reasoning occur is central to their effectiveness (Darling & Steinberg, 1993). Thus parenting practices take on different meanings, depending on whether they are accompanied by warmth or by hostility. The correlation between physical punishment and externalizing problems, for example, is greater when mothers are low in warmth than when they are high in warmth (McLoyd & Smith, 2002; Simons, Wu, Lin, Gordon, & Conger, 2000). When control is accompanied by warmth, it has fewer negative effects than it does in the context of rejection and hostility (Brody & Flor, 1998; Kilgore, Snyder, & Lentz, 2000; Lansford et al., 2010). Presumably, warmth and acceptance indicate a parent's love or concern, and so control is less threatening to a child's sense of autonomy. As well, warmth and acceptance are more likely to foster a desire to please the parent. In this way, reactance (or resistance to the parent's wishes) is lessened, and conformity with parental dictates is facilitated.

### Cultural Context

There is considerable evidence that the negative impact of authoritarian parenting found for Western European individuals is not so evident for those from other cultural settings. This includes individuals from different ethnic groups within Western countries (e.g., Deater-Deckard, Dodge, Bates, & Pettit, 1996; Lamborn, Dornbusch, & Steinberg, 1996), from different countries of origin (e.g., Chao, 2001; Lansford et al., 2005), and sometimes also from different religious backgrounds (e.g., Gunnoe, Hetherington, & Reiss, 2006; Ellison, Musick, & Holden, 2011). In all these cases, the detrimental effects of harsh parenting on middle-class children of Western European heritage do not appear, and may even be associated with better outcomes (Chao, 2001). One explanation is that authoritarian parenting takes on a different meaning as a function of cultural or parental beliefs. Thus Rudy and Grusec (2001, 2006) compared the correlates of authoritarian parenting in a Middle Eastern Canadian sample and a sample of Western European Canadians. Strict, authoritarian parenting was linked to more negative perceptions of the child and reduced warmth, but only in the case of Western Europeans. The importance of parental beliefs is further underlined in the finding that spanking was related to children's depression when mothers did not endorse it as an appropriate form of discipline, but not when it was seen as the proper way to discipline (McLoyd, Kaplan, Hardaway, & Wood, 2007). In the first case, mothers who spanked presumably did so because they were angry and had lost control; in the second case, mothers meant it as a teaching device.

## Do Different Forms of Reasoning and Different Forms of Power Assertion Have Similar Outcomes?

*Reasoning*

Already noted is the fact that different forms of reasoning have different outcomes. Other-oriented reasoning is deemed to be particularly effective because it arouses empathy for the person harmed (Hoffman, 1970b). And children are more responsive when they are told that sharing will make the recipient happy than when they are told it is good to share (Eisenberg-Berg & Geisheker, 1979). Reasons need to be appropriate to the domain of the misdeed: What works for moral transgressions or harm to others does not work for social conventional transgressions, which are not inherently bad or immoral.

*Physical Punishment: Is Spanking Harmful?*
*What about Other Forms of Power Assertion?*

The impact of different forms of punishment on children, particularly that of physical or corporal punishment, has attracted substantial attention from both parents and makers of social policy. A definition of corporal punishment, provided by the United Nations Committee on the Rights of the Child, appears in Table 5.2.

Opponents of the use of physical punishment point out that adults have a right not to be physically assaulted, and they argue that children should be granted the same right. Negative views of physical punishment (specifically, punishment intended to inflict pain) have led to its being declared illegal in approximately 50 countries at this writing. These countries include Sweden, Finland, Germany, Romania, Israel, New Zealand, Tunisia, and Peru. Notably absent from the list are the United States and Canada. Corporal punishment is not outlawed in the United States, and Holden (2002) suggests that it is highly unlikely that it will be, given the importance placed in American history on corporal punishment as part of childrearing. Also, American beliefs about the privacy of the family and personal freedoms discourage societal and governmental intervention in aspects of family life. The situation in Canada is somewhat different. In 2004, Canada's Supreme Court upheld a provision of the Criminal Code that allowed teachers, parents, and legal guardians to use reasonable force to correct children in their charge. It laid out guidelines for reasonable force, declaring that corporal punishment must be "by way of correction" and that a child must be capable of benefiting from the correction (i.e., between the ages of 2 and 12 years). It must not result in bodily harm or leave a mark that

---

**TABLE 5.2. United Nations Statement on Corporal Punishment and Other Forms of Cruel Punishment**

The United Nations Committee on the Rights of the Child has defined corporal punishment in these words (reproduced at *http://hrlibrary.umn. edu/crc/comment8.html*):

> . . . any punishment in which physical force is used and intended to cause some degree of pain or discomfort, however light. Most involves hitting ("smacking", "slapping", "spanking") children, with the hand or with an implement—a whip, stick, belt, shoe, wooden spoon, etc. But it can also involve, for example, kicking, shaking or throwing children, scratching, pinching, biting, pulling hair or boxing ears, forcing children to stay in uncomfortable positions, burning, scalding or forced ingestion (for example, washing children's mouths out with soap or forcing them to swallow hot spices). In the view of the Committee, corporal punishment is invariably degrading. In addition, there are other non-physical forms of punishment which are also cruel and degrading and thus incompatible with the Convention. These include, for example, punishment which belittles, humiliates, denigrates, scapegoats, threatens, scares or ridicules the child.

lasts for several hours, and must be administered with a bare hand. For many parents in the United States and Canada at least, corporal punishment is seen as an acceptable intervention. More than 70% of Americans agreed in 2012 that "it is sometimes necessary to discipline a child with a good, hard spanking" (Smith, Marsden, Hout, & Kim, 2013). In Canada, 48% of mothers reported that they had used physical punishment in a mild form (smacking, slapping, pinching) in the past year (Oldershaw, 2002).

Aside from the philosophical argument involving the rights of children, there is the important question of whether or not physical punishment is even effective. Opponents argue that it is a predictor of later antisocial behavior and a potential way station to physical abuse (Strassburg, Dodge, Pettit, & Bates, 1994; Straus, 1996). Supporters see occasional mild corporal punishment (spanking of a child's extremities with an open hand) —used only between toddlerhood and puberty, and used in the context of authoritative parenting—as a useful social-ization tool (Baumrind & Thompson, 2002; Baumrind, Larzelere, & Cowan, 2002) and one that young children accept as a reasonable and fair parental practice (Helwig et al., 2014; Siegal & Barclay, 1985). Pro-ponents have also pointed out that much of the research linking corpo-ral punishment and externalizing problems is correlational (although that has changed in recent years). As well, there has been a general failure to separate harsh and abusive physical punishment from mild forms, or to distinguish the impact of corporal punishment on very young children from its impact on adolescents. Thus the argument is that many of the studies cited by the critics of corporal punishment are open to different interpretations.

### RESEARCH EVIDENCE

So what does the research actually indicate? First of all, there is evi-dence that corporal punishment and physical abuse are not causally related. The two are correlated (Gershoff, 2002), and statistics with respect to child homicide rates suggest a link between favorable atti-tudes toward corporal punishment and extreme physical abuse (World Health Organization, 2002). Parents who have spanked their children at 1 year of age are more likely to be involved with child protection services in ensuing years (S. J. Lee, Grogan-Kaylor, & Berger, 2014). However, evidence from behavior genetic studies suggests that the use of corporal punishment does not make it more likely that parents will become physically abusive. Shared genetic influences account for a substantial part of the correlation between parents' use of corporal punishment and children's antisocial behavior, whereas they do not account for that between parents' physical abuse and children's antisocial behavior (Jaffee et al., 2004). Thus corporal punishment and child abuse, although correlated, appear to have different origins: Corporal punishment is more likely to have its roots in features of the child, and abusive parenting is more likely to have its roots in features of the family environment and characteristics of the abusive parent.

Other studies have pointed to the importance of context in determining the impact of physical punishment. Physical punishment has adverse effects on European American children but not African American children, for whom it is actually associated with *lower* levels of externalizing problems (Lansford, Deater-Deckard, Dodge, Bates, & Pettit, 2004). One explanation is that physical punishment is more normative in African American families, and that therefore it may be perceived simply as a fair and appropriate practice (rather than, for example, a loss of self-control on a parent's part). In a test of this hypothesis, Lansford et al. (2005) assessed the relation between physical punishment and children's aggression and anxiety in six countries that differed in how frequently, based on interviews with children and mothers, physical punishment was employed. The countries, in order of physical punishment usage from least to most, were Thailand, China, the Philippines, Italy, India, and Kenya. Lansford et al. found, as they had expected, that countries with the lowest use of physical discipline showed the strongest association between mothers' use of physical punishment and children's behavior problems. However, they also found in all countries, regardless of the normativeness of physical punishment, that greater use of physical discipline was associated with more externalizing and internalizing problems. In a later study, Lansford et al. (2010) found that children's perceptions of their mothers' behavior as rejecting mediated between physical punishment and their aggression and anxiety. The conclusion, then, is that when children perceive harsh punishment as a sign of rejection, it will have negative effects on their well-being. The meaning children attach to their parents' behavior is important in understanding the impact of harsh forms of parenting.

A meta-analysis by Gershoff and Grogan-Kaylor (2016) included a large number of longitudinal studies; it also distinguished between physical abuse and physical punishment in the form of spanking or hitting on the buttocks or extremities with an open hand. In all, Gershoff and Grogan-Kaylor reviewed 75 studies that included 160,927 children from 13 countries (a reflection of the considerable interest in this aspect of parenting). The results of their meta-analysis yielded substantial support for the position that physical punishment does lead to externalizing problems. Indeed, this is hardly a surprising outcome—given that parents who use some form of physical force to get their way are, at the same time, modeling physical force as a way of resolving conflicts in general.

### Do Other Forms of Power Assertion Have Negative Consequences?

Although physical punishment has received most attention with respect to its impact on socialization, there are many other forms of power assertion that may, or may not, have similar negative consequences for children's behavior. Note in Table 5.2, for example, that the United Nations Committee on the Rights of the Child refers to the existence of forms of punishment beyond corporal punishment that are also cruel and degrading. These include punishment that belittles, humiliates, denigrates, scapegoats, threatens, scares, or ridicules. Research evidence exists for the effects of some of these other forms. For example, adolescents rate yelling as less fair than talking (Padilla-Walker & Carlo, 2004).

Gershoff et al. (2010) compared forms of power assertion and their relation to aggression and anxiety in six different countries. They found that physical punishment, yelling, scolding, and the expression of disappointment were associated with higher levels of aggression. Time out, teaching about good and bad behavior, getting children to apologize, taking away privileges, shaming, withdrawing love, threatening punishment, and promising treats or privileges were not associated either positively or negatively with aggression. Positive associations with anxiety were found for physical punishment, expressing disappointment, time out, and shaming. Failure to find any beneficial effects of power assertion, of course, underlines the important role played by reasoning in association with power assertion.

## ■ EFFECTIVE PARENTING IN THE CONTROL DOMAIN: CORE SKILLS

In general terms, effective parenting in the control domain requires that parents use modest levels of power assertion, along with explanation for why a particular action is undesirable. The value being transmitted must be clear and consistently enforced. Both punishment and reasoning must be appropriately matched to the misdeed, as well as to characteristics of the child such as temperament and age. Finally, the child must see the parenting intervention as a sign of parental caring and not of parental rejection.

One way of organizing effective parenting in the control domain is to think of parenting in that domain as involving core skills. These core skills include (1) knowing a child well enough to be able to select approaches that would be seen by that particular child as acceptable and convincing; (2) taking the child's perspective in the specific situation, so that an intervention that is appropriate at that particular point in time can be selected; (3) making rules clear and consistent; (4) supporting the child's sense of autonomy; (5) accepting the child; and (6) making the discipline appropriate to the misdeed. I discuss each of these in turn.

### Knowledge

It is important for agents of socialization to select disciplinary responses that are suitable for a specific child in the current situation. Parents who are knowledgeable about children's views and how they are likely to react can tailor their interventions in a way that is more likely to achieve success (Grusec, Goodnow, & Kuczynski, 2000). Whether or not rules are understood, whether a particular form of discipline is seen as fair, whether an intervention is perceived to be a reflection of caring rather than hostility, and whether a highly power-assertive strategy is seen to indicate importance to the parent (as opposed to an angry and irrational outburst) are all useful pieces of information for a parent to have in the task of value learning and behavior control.

A number of studies have shown the importance of knowledge in the discipline process. One of these (Hastings & Grusec, 1997), for example, found that parents who knew what their adolescents reported they were thinking and feeling during a past parent–child conflict expressed greater satisfaction with the outcome of the conflict (in the case of mothers) and had fewer conflicts (in the case of fathers). Another study (Davidov & Grusec, 2006b) found that mothers who were more knowledgeable about their children's evaluations of different discipline strategies were more likely to have children who, after initial resistance, complied with their request to tidy a playroom; this compliance was accomplished through their responsive, and apparently knowledgeable, reactions to the resistance.

There are a number of ways in which parents can become more knowledgeable about or better able to predict their children's reactions in a discipline situation. Careful observation, questioning about thoughts and feelings, and encouragement of communication are among them. Not surprisingly, parents who have more accurate knowledge of their children's views of discipline also report more authoritative parenting practices and fewer authoritarian or permissive practices (Davidov, Grusec, & Wolfe, 2012).

## Perspective Taking

Trying to understand how situations look from the other person's point of view is a positive approach for any social interaction, especially when conflict is involved. This is certainly true in the case of parenting. A parent, by taking a child's perspective, will have a better chance of identifying extenuating circumstances or misunderstandings, and therefore of adopting an intervention that will gain successful compliance. In one study (Lundell, Grusec, McShane, & Davidov, 2008), for example, older adolescents were asked to talk about recent disagreements they had had with their mothers and what they hoped to accomplish during those disagreements. Those with mothers who were high in perspective taking were more likely to cite compromise as their desired outcome, as opposed to wanting their mothers to change their minds or to feel bad. Accordingly, maternal perspective taking was associated with less intense conflict. And in a study of young adolescents, mothers who reported they were more likely to take their children's perspective in difficult situations became increasingly autonomy-supportive over the course of 2 years (Mageau, Sherman, Grusec, Koestner, & Bureau, 2016). These sorts of results, then, suggest that perspective taking can lead not only to more optimal approaches to discipline, but to a more positive context or climate in which socialization can take place.

## Consistency

Rules and expectations with respect to appropriate behavior need to be clearly laid out and consistently enforced. Inconsistent discipline at an early age predicts behavioral problems at a later time (Loeber, Green, Keenan, & Lahey, 1995; Manongdo & Ramírez García, 2011; Tildesley & Andrews, 2008). One way it does this is by encouraging positive attitudes toward delinquent or antisocial behavior (Halgunseth, Perkins, Lippold, & Nix, 2013). Thus parents' inconsistent enforcement of rules indicates to their children that standards of conduct are ambiguous. Inconsistent discipline also encourages children to morally disengage from antisocial behavior by applying self-exonerating justifications or reconstructing antisocial acts so they seem less wrong (Bandura, 1999). Finally, of course, parental inconsistency may simply encourage children to engage in antisocial acts with the hope and reasonable expectation that they will not be punished.

## Autonomy Support

Autonomy support includes providing meaningful rationales for compliance with parental requests and demands, providing choice and opportunities for taking initiative within the limits of those demands, and acknowledging children's feelings. This approach is associated with the internalization of values. Parenting that is pressuring, coercive, or intrusive, and that includes guilt induction, conditional regard (criticism of a child rather than of the child's act), and threats of punishment, predicts externalizing and internalizing problems in both children and adolescents (Joussemet, Landry, & Koestner, 2008).

Not only is coercive control associated with lack of freely given compliance, but it has also been shown to lead to reactance, or the desire to do just the opposite of what has been requested (Brehm & Brehm, 1981). Van Petegem, Soenens, Vansteenkiste, and Beyers (2015), for example, found that coercive parental control was associated with frustration of needs for autonomy or a feeling of being pressured. Frustration of the need for autonomy predicted reactance, which was associated with externalizing problems and noncompliance, as well as internalizing problems. Van Petegem et al. suggest that reactance produces internalizing problems, in addition to externalizing ones, because feeling compelled to do the opposite of what is requested is also challenging to autonomy and therefore produces anxiety and depression.

The Van Petegem et al. study also demonstrated the independence of control and rule setting; the latter was unrelated to autonomy need frustration, reactance, or problematic behavior. Rules can be followed happily, so long as they are not applied in an intrusive and coercive way.

## Acceptance

There is considerable evidence that parental rejection has a negative impact on children's development: Maladjustment is more frequent among individuals who report that their parenting was rejecting rather than accepting (Rohner & Britner, 2002). It could be argued, of course, that the relation between rejection and behavioral problems is simply a reflection of the fact that parents and children are genetically similar, and that disagreeable or problem parents have disagreeable or problem children. However, the relation between rejecting parenting and problem outcomes holds for both biologically related children and their mothers and adopted children and their mothers (Deater-Deckard, Ivy, & Petrill, 2006), so genetic similarity cannot be the sole explanation. One of the ways in which rejection impairs positive socioemotional functioning is by affecting children's ability to deal with stress. Thus high levels of parental rejection adversely affect the development and subsequent functioning of neurobiological systems responsible for the regulation of stress and negative emotion (Gunnar, 2000).

As discussed earlier in this chapter, the emotional context in which parenting occurs, as well as having a direct effect on child development, also moderates the relation between parenting and children's social and emotional development. The quality of the parent–child relationship, as reflected in indications of acceptance, warmth, and caring, affects the way in which parenting of a harsh nature is perceived or interpreted. In positive relationships, for example, harshness may be seen as an indication of concern for a child's well-being, whereas in negative relationships it may promote feelings of anger.

## Employment of Appropriate Consequences

There is no all-purpose response to all misdeeds. Punishment needs to fit the crime—a fit presumably mediated by children's view of the fairness of a control strategy, given the nature of the rule that has been broken (Grusec & Goodnow, 1994). Reasons need to be appropriate to the domain of the misdeed they follow (Killen, Breton, Ferguson, & Handler, 1994; Nucci, 1984). Thus failing to raise one's hand in the classroom before speaking, or stepping out of line, is better addressed by discussions about maintaining order than by discussions about how such actions might affect the welfare of others. Children and adolescents also have views about the way in which discipline is administered; adolescents find maternal yelling, for example, inappropriate in response to violations of social conventions, but not in response to moral violations (Padilla-Walker, 2008).

## ■ OTHER PARENTING STRATEGIES IN THE CONTROL DOMAIN

Discipline is not the only way that parents control or modify their children's behavior. They also reward good behavior in an attempt to increase its frequency. They avoid actions that end up rewarding bad behavior. And they monitor children's behavior, as well as encouraging children to talk about their activities—two means of gaining information about whether or not their children are behaving antisocially, so that they can, if necessary and possible, intervene.

### Reward

Although one would expect that parents would make ample use of reinforcement for socializing their children, there were few examples of this in the narratives collected in my lab. Here is one of the rare ones:

> "I won a swimming competition when I thought i would totally lose it. My father was so happy of this and so proud of me. (he was there and actually helped me get out of the water and while doing that he was extremely happy and proud of me and kept saying 'you did it'). I learned to believe in myself and my abilities." (Male, age 12, Middle Eastern)

#### *Undermining Intrinsic Motivation*

Just as power assertion has its challenges and difficulties, so too does reward. Self-determination theorists have written extensively about how reward that is contingent on performance of an inherently interesting action undermines interest in that activity. A love of learning, for example, can be spoiled when stickers and praise are given for good performance (Deci, Koestner, & Ryan, 1999). The harmful impact of reward on intrinsic motivation was demonstrated in an early study where preschoolers were observed as they spent considerable time at a drawing table in the nursery school. When some of the children were told they would receive a reward for drawing pictures, they began to spend less time at the drawing table. This decrease in interest did not occur in the case of children who were not promised a reward (Lepper, Greene, & Nisbett, 1973).

## Conditional Positive Regard

Social rewards in the form of conditional positive regard (increased levels of attention and approval on the parent's part when the child has behaved well) have also been shown to have a negative impact on children's and young adults' desire or motivation for acceptable behavior (Assor, Roth, & Deci, 2004; Roth, 2008). Roth, Assor, Niemiec, Ryan, and Deci (2009) compared the effects of conditional positive regard and conditional negative regard (withdrawing attention and affection) in response to children's actions. In the positive condition, parents provided more affection than usual; in the negative condition, they provided less affection than usual. An example from their study of conditional positive regard was "I feel that when I'm studying hard, my father appreciates me much more than usual." An example of negative conditional regard was "If I do poorly in school, my mother will ignore me for a while." Although positive conditional regard would seem to be a preferred method for socializing children, Roth et al. found that both positive and negative regard had an adverse impact on adolescents' performance in school as well as on their emotion control. Conditional positive regard was associated with feelings of "internal compulsion" (i.e., introjected rather than internalized motivation), and this, in turn, was associated with problems in emotion control as well as teachers' lower ratings of how much interest, enjoyment, and curiosity in studying the adolescents displayed, as opposed to being focused on tests and grades. Not surprisingly, in the case of conditional negative regard, resentment toward the parents was one outcome, in addition to undermining of the capacity for school engagement and emotion regulation. What *does* work, then, to encourage interest in desirable activities? Assor et al. found that autonomy support—taking a child's perspective and providing a reason or explanation for why a particular behavior was desirable—was a predictor of positive outcomes.

## Effectiveness of Praise as a Function of Attribution, Target, and Context

Research underlining the negative consequences of conditional positive regard does not mean that reward or praise is never effective in modifying behavior. A considerable body of research has shown that attributing children's achievement to relatively invariant factors such as ability ("You're very smart") impairs their performance in subsequent challenging situations. On the other hand, attribution of achievement to more readily modifiable factors such as effort ("You tried really hard") produces "mastery-oriented" individuals and is associated with maintenance or improvements in performance following failure (e.g., Dweck, 1975; Dweck & Reppucci, 1973; Weiner, 1974).

A different picture with respect to praising persons emerges in work with prosocial behavior as the outcome. Thus Miller, Brickman, and Bolen (1975) found that telling children that they were neat and tidy—that is, attributing a positive characteristic to the actors—was more effective at reducing littering on the playground than telling them that they *ought* to be neat and tidy. In another study, Grusec and Redler (1980) encouraged children who had just played a game to share their winnings from that game with poor children, and either praised them for their behavior or told them that they must have donated because they were helpful people. Those who had been told that they were helpful people were more likely to help another adult a week later, and more likely to collect art material and make drawings for hospitalized children a week or so after that, than were those who had been praised. The effect was strongest for children ages 7 and 8 years; the two conditions were identical in their effect on prosocial behavior for 10-year-olds.

SUMMARY ▪ ▪ ▪ ▪ ▪ ▪ ▪ ▪ ▪ ▪ ▪ ▪ ▪ ▪ ▪ ▪ ▪ ▪ ▪ ▪ ▪ ▪ ▪ ▪ ▪ ▪ ▪ ▪ ▪ ▪ ▪ ▪ ▪ ▪ ▪

The picture with respect to reward, then, is complex, not unlike that with respect to power assertion. Outcomes appear to depend on the nature of the reward, the age of the child, and the behavior of interest. At this point, developmental psychologists probably know more about power assertion than they do about reward. One thing is evident, however: Care needs to be taken with the use of reward (as, indeed, is the case with power assertion).

## Negative Reinforcement

No discussion of control is complete without reference to the work of Gerald Patterson and his colleagues (e.g., Patterson, 1980; Snyder, Reid, & Patterson, 2003). Coercion theory, as developed by these research-ers, emerged from a behavior modification perspective and therefore had little to say about concepts such as internalization and attributions. Indeed, Patterson (1997) argues that positive actions become automatic simply as a result of constant repetition. In research on family dynam-ics and aggressive behavior, Patterson (1980) demonstrated how moth-ers in distressed families inadvertently reinforce children's (particu-larly boys') difficult behavior. In a typical instance, a mother makes a request for a specific behavior, and her child responds with resistance to the request or even anger. The mother in turn escalates her behavior, becoming angry and hostile. This reaction leads to an increased nega-tive reaction on the part of the child until the mother finally gives up: Her child has won, and she retreats. In this way, the child's aggressive noncompliance is reinforced by the withdrawal of an aversive event—the mother's ceasing to nag. Importantly, other members of the family do not react in the same way. Other children do not give in so easily to their sibling's aversive behavior, and so they keep the exchange going. And fathers remain relatively uninvolved, assuming the role of resident "guests." Mothers are the crisis managers; hence the title of Patterson's 1980 monograph, "Mothers: The Unacknowledged Victims." Once a pattern of coercive interaction has been established in the family, it car-ries over into interactions outside the family. Through a developmental cascade of arrested social and academic skills and decreased opportuni-ties for prosocial learning, children with conduct problems turn into antisocial adolescents (Dishion, Véronneau, & Myers, 2010).

One very valuable feature of Patterson's work is his microanaly-sis of family interactions. We know, in general terms, that harsh and inconsistent parenting promotes antisocial and aggressive behavior. However, what the careful observation of family interactions does is to show one way in which harsh and inconsistent parenting is actu-ally carried out and how it affects children's behavior through par-enting that is less than ideal. The interactive nature of socialization is once again made clear: In the present case, a difficult child drives a marginally competent socializing agent to inadvertently strengthen aversive behavior by cyclical reactions of withdrawal and giving in. Intervention studies have provided further support for the coercion model by showing that programs targeting coercive parenting practices reduce children's conduct problems (Dishion, Patterson, & Kavanaugh, 1992).

## Monitoring

Monitoring, a form of behavioral control that involves attempts by various means to know what children are doing, enables parents to keep track of their children's activities—how they spend their time when not with their parents, who their friends are, how well they are doing at school—while allowing those children to have greater autonomy. It is a strategy that requires close surveillance and includes asking children themselves for information, as well as seeking information from teachers, peers, and other parents (Crouter, Helms-Erikson, Updegraff, & McHale, 1999). Reasonable levels of monitoring that are not overly controlling and are carried out in the context of a positive parent–child relationship have been shown to predict positive child behavior (Fletcher, Steinberg, & Williams-Wheeler, 2004; Soenens, Vansteenkiste, Luyckx, & Goossens, 2006; Waizenhofer, Buchanan, & Jackson-Newsom, 2004). And in a meta-analysis of studies of the relation between various forms of parenting and delinquency, Hoeve et al. (2009) found strong linkages between low levels of active monitoring and antisocial behavior.

## Disclosure

As children move into early adolescence, their increasing independence allows them to spend greater amounts of time away from their parents' observation and supervision (Dijkstra & Veenstra, 2011; Larson, 2001). Opportunities for knowledge of how their children are thinking and feeling and what they are doing are therefore reduced for parents, and so at least some of their major socialization tools are lost. Alternative methods of gaining knowledge have to be acquired. One of these is disclosure.

Kerr and Stattin (2000) and Stattin and Kerr (2000), in two influential papers, found that adolescents' spontaneous disclosure of information was a better predictor of their positive outcomes than either solicitation of information or control of their activities. Not surprisingly, the relation between disclosure and adolescent behavior has been shown to be bidirectional, with children who disclose becoming less antisocial, and children who are antisocial becoming less likely to disclose (Kerr, Stattin, & Burk, 2010).

Disclosure does not mean that socialization has somehow been transferred to the adolescent. Although disclosure gives adolescents the power to manage the amount of information parents have, it is facilitated by parenting. Parenting style, acceptance of a child's perspective, responsiveness, behavior control, autonomy support, and a mother's own disclosure have all been linked to adolescent disclosure (Chaparro & Grusec, 2015; Darling, Cumsille, Caldwell, & Dowdy, 2006; Mageau et al., 2017; Smetana, Metzger, Gettman, & Campione-Barr, 2006; Soenens et al., 2006). Adolescents report that negative reactions such as showing mistrust, acting sad or disappointed, and lecturing in response to disclosure are responses that inhibit it (Tokić & Pećnik, 2011).

Among the reasons adolescents offer for disclosing information to their parents are to seek advice and to feel better (Chaparro & Grusec, 2015). Adolescents feel more obligated to disclose in areas where they believe their parents have legitimate authority to intervene, such as health and well-being (Smetana, Villalobos, Tasopoulos-Chan, Gettman, & Campione-Barr, 2007). Failure to disclose is also different from secrecy or a deliberate attempt to hide information. Thus the two have different correlates, with failure to disclose associated with lower levels of maternal authoritativeness, and secrecy with mothers' dispositional tendency toward anger (Almas, Grusec, & Tackett, 2011). Adolescents also distinguish between telling parents only if asked, as opposed to concealing information. The former is associated with better family relationships and adjustment, whereas concealment is associated with adverse outcomes. These adverse outcomes are less serious, however, when they are associated with acts of omission such as leaving out details and avoidance as opposed to outright lying (Laird & Marrero, 2010; Marshall, Tilton-Weaver, & Bosdet, 2005).

## ■ CONCLUSION

The considerable attention paid by researchers to the topic of discipline and other forms of behavior management reflects the intense interest of parents, as well as of mental health professionals. A general conclusion is that discipline works best when its level and nature are appropriate, when it is combined with clear and reasonable rules, and when it is administered in a context of perceived parental caring as well as of autonomy support. Rewards of a material and social nature can be useful under certain conditions to encourage positive behavior, but can have serious drawbacks. Giving in to children's aversive behavior or withdrawing from conflict situations is particularly detrimental to the socialization process. Finally, knowledge of children's thoughts and activities is central and can be obtained either from children themselves, from other people in their environment, or by providing conditions that encourage voluntary disclosure.

Children's antisocial behavior, along with their distress, is an event that is demanding of parental action. Less demanding of response are the two domains that I address in Chapters 6 and 7. Teaching children about values and ensuring that they are exposed to positive social behavior are strategies that can have a significant impact on children's socialization. They require more conscious effort on the part of parents, however, because opportunities for their use can be easily ignored.

## CHAPTER 1 SCENARIOS REVISITED

The two scenarios presented in Chapter 1 as examples of the control domain are reproduced in Box 5.1, along with possible responses on the parents' part.

In the first scenario, Alternative A, determining whether Amanda is getting enough sleep, would be an excellent place to start. Is Amanda watching TV or playing video games too late into the evening? If so, should these activities be rationed? Alternative B, looking together for a solution to the problem, is a good one to add. Done in a collaborative way rather than a dictatorial one, it provides a good example of autonomy support. Alternative C, punishing Amanda for not getting up in the morning by deducting money from her allowance, is a possible response but could be less desirable from the standpoint of providing autonomy support. If it were seen by Amanda as a sign of caring on her parents' part, that would be helpful.

In the second scenario, Alternative A, where Charlie's mother expresses her disappointment in him, is an example of psychological control—a strategy that has been linked to negative outcomes. Alternative B is interesting because it is other-oriented and focuses Charlie's attention on the harm he has done to his brother, as well as offering him a way of alleviating that harm. Alternative C assumes that Charlie does not like spending time in his room and that his mother knows this; should this be the case, it could also be an effective strategy.

**BOX 5.1.** Scenarios from the Control Domain

*Amanda (8 years old) is extremely difficult to get up in the morning. As a result, she makes other people late for work or school.*

A. Her parents make sure Amanda is getting enough sleep.

B. Her parents sit down with Amanda and they all talk about what they and she can do to help her get up in the morning.

C. Her parents deduct money from her allowance for each morning Amanda doesn't get up.

*Charlie (14 years old) is frustrated because he can't solve a math problem for school. His mother is trying to help him when his younger brother asks if he can borrow Charlie's new baseball bat. Charlie yells at his brother and tells him to keep his grubby hands off his (Charlie's) possessions.*

A. Mom says she is very upset and disappointed by Charlie's behavior.

B. Mom suggests that Charlie apologize to his brother.

C. Mom tells Charlie to go to his room until he can control his temper.

# CHAPTER 6

# Learning Values in the Guided Learning Domain

## *Conversations and Reminiscences about Values*

In the control domain, children act either in an antisocial way that violates social norms, or in a prosocial way that accords with social norms. In the former case, they may be disciplined; in the latter, they may be rewarded. In the guided learning domain, the socialization process is quite different. It does not involve a response to specific actions that are antisocial or prosocial in nature and that require immediate attention. It occurs, instead, when caregivers use special moments as opportunities to teach. These moments can include taking an opportunity to tell or read a story, or to comment on a current event where there is a lesson to be learned, or to respond to someone's question, or to help someone learn a new social behavior. Socialization in the guided learning domain also occurs in the context of reminiscence, when children and parents have conversations about events that happened at some earlier point in time but that may still provide an opportunity for teaching.

From an evolutionary perspective, guided learning is a very useful way of helping children construct an understanding of values and positive social behavior. Humans have evolved with a set of adaptations that enables them to learn from and with others, including immaturity at birth, a long period of dependence, and considerable intellectual ability. Because of the learning opportunities provided by these adaptations, they are in a good position to benefit from continued interactions with experienced group members who can teach them what they need to know in order to survive and flourish (Gauvain & Perez, 2015). Language ability, of course, is central to this learning.

## ■ THE ZONE OF PROXIMAL DEVELOPMENT, AND SCAFFOLDING

Developmental psychologists have had a long-standing interest in guided learning and its role in children's development, particularly their cognitive development. Piaget (1936) argued that if children are to know something, they have to construct that knowledge themselves. However, the Russian psychologist Lev Vygotsky (e.g., 1978) adopted a different view by arguing that cognitive growth occurs in a social context, and that this social context has an effect on the form that knowledge takes. Thus many of children's cognitive skills emerge from social interactions with others who are more competent, including parents, teachers, and older siblings. Children's discoveries, then, come out of cooperative or collaborative dialogues with those who have greater knowledge.

Conversation or dialogue must take place in what Vygotsky referred to as the "zone of proximal development." This zone marks the boundary between what a child can do independently and what the child can do with guidance from a teacher or more skilled partner. In Vygotsky's (1978) words, it is "the distance between the actual developmental level as determined by independent problem solving and the level of potential development as determined through problem solving under adult guidance, or in collaboration with more capable peers" (p. 86). The zone of proximal development, of course, is always shifting: Once children have expanded their knowledge base, their developmental level expands, and the zone of proximal development is raised to a new level. Key to the whole teaching and learning process is internalization, whereby an operation that initially requires external support is continuously modified until it is internalized or generated independent of this external support. In other words, when discussions are conducted appropriately, parent and child reach a shared understanding as the parent's position is internalized or taken over as the child's own (Puntambekar & Hubscher, 2005).

Wood, Bruner, and Ross (1976) introduced the idea of "scaffolding" to explain successful teaching: A teacher working in the zone of proximal development needs to scaffold the learning process. As the student becomes more proficient, assistance is gradually decreased, so that the responsibility for learning is shifted from teacher to student. Once the student has made use of the scaffolding to master the task at hand, the scaffolding can be removed, and the student will then be able to complete the task independently. In a demonstration of scaffolding, Wood and Middleton (1975) found that mothers supported the learning of a new task by providing general encouragement, setting out specific instructions, or directly demonstrating correct actions. They suggested that no one of these strategies works best for learning. Rather, the effective teaching approach is to vary the strategy as a reflection of how well a child is learning. When children are doing well, teachers become less specific in their help. And when children are beginning to struggle, increasingly specific instructions are given until progress is occurring once again. There is considerable evidence that scaffolding and conversation are important determinants of children's cognitive development. As an example, Bernier, Carlson, and Whipple (2010) found that maternal scaffolding, sensitive responding, and attention to children's inner mental states or "mind-mindedness" (Meins et al., 2003) when the children were 12–15 months old predicted their executive functioning at 18–26 months of age.

## Guided Learning and Moral Reasoning

Early research on guided learning in the area of moral development focused on changing children's level of moral reasoning. The premise was that exposure to a higher stage of moral reasoning challenges a child's current thinking and thereby produces a state of disequilibrium. When in this state, children experience cognitive conflict that leads to questioning of their current way of thinking, and this experience encourages more equilibrated or higher-level reasoning. Studies clearly indicated that the discrepancy between two individuals involved in a moral discussion should not be too great—that is, not outside the zone of proximal development (Berkowitz, Gibbs, & Broughton, 1980; Taylor & Walker, 1997).

A different approach to scaffolding the development of moral reasoning emerges from a study by Walker, Hennig, and Krettenauer (2000). These investigators were interested in comparing the nature of discussions about moral reasoning by parents and by peers. Recall Piaget's belief that parents have a less important role to play in moral development than do peers, because parents are authority figures and therefore provide fewer opportunities for stimulating moral growth. Walker et al. wanted to find out if conversations with peers were, in fact, more effective in increasing children's level of moral reasoning than were conversations with parents. What they found was that moral development was affected by both peer and parent discussions. For both peer and parent groups, reflecting on or restating the other's point of view led to higher levels of moral reasoning than did critiquing the other's point of view. In contrast, devaluing the task and expressing hostility were detrimental when they came from parents, but had positive effects when they came from peers. This latter finding, Walker and colleagues suggested, may be an indication that children are better able to tolerate hostility from their peers than from their parents. Interestingly, Walker et al. found that informative discussions that involved the sharing of opinions and that included discussion of agreements, disagreements, and requests for change were not effective, possibly because they were interpreted as opinionated lecturing.

## ■ CONVERSATIONS ABOUT VALUES AND COPING

At the beginning of this chapter, I have noted that guided learning can occur either when a parent and child are discussing principles and behavior that are not linked to any specific thing the child has done, or when parent and child are reminiscing about past events in which the child has been an actor. Talking about the child's specific past experiences would seem to put the interaction into another domain—control in the case of antisocial or prosocial events, and protection in the case of distress regulation. Reminiscence has a different flavor, however, that moves it into the guided learning domain. More than listening to rationales for positive behavior in the midst of an emotional situation, or being reassured in a distressing situation, joint discussion or reminiscence about past events and the accompanying reflection allow parent and child some distance from the event in question. The experiences are less immediate and more integrated into the child's sense of history, and thus negative thoughts or feelings are not as likely to be present. Conversation at a later point in time, when there has been a cooling-off period (in the case of antisocial behavior) or a reduction in distress, also allows for the formation of new points of view, knowledge, and understanding. Emotions may arise in these conversations, but they can be dealt with more easily in a less fraught context (Wainryb & Recchia, 2014).

I begin the discussion by considering conversations that do not involve reflecting on a child's past behavior, and then move on in a later section to those that do. In the case of the former—conversations that are not about the individual's past actions—I include storytelling, discussions about positive social values and actions, and discussions that arise in response to children's questions or observations.

## Storytelling and Socialization of Values

Here are narratives from our lab that involve the guided learning domain and, specifically, the use of stories to teach values. Again, the sex and ethnicity of each narrator are indicated, along with age at the time he or she learned the value.

"This value was taught to me through a Chinese poem. It is a very famous poem and probably one of the first to be taught to children in China. The poem describes a farmer out in the field in the middle of the day, the sun is shining, and he is sweating. It ends with the question, loosely translated: 'Who appreciates that the food in our plates came with such hard work and labour?' While in Chinese school, this was one of the poems we were supposed to learn and memorize. My mom told me the meaning of the poem, and through it, taught me not to waste or take things for granted." (Female, age 11, East Asian)

"My teacher asked me to read a book The monk who sold his Ferrari and this book was really interesting it had a lot of moral stuff in it, one of which was helping others and the book was really effective in teaching how you should spend your life, etc." (Female, age 15, Western European)

"My mother always told me to help others in need. She used to read me books from Iran that contained several fables. She read me one story every night after dinner and then would proceed to explaining to me why the moral that was taught in the story was important. One particular story was about a colony of ants who worked hard in the summer to gather food and supplies so that they would survive in the winter. However there was a grasshopper who would always mock them and tell them to put their work off until later, because they were wasting their summer doing hard work. The ants of course did not listen. Winter came around and the ants had all the food and supplies they needed to survive, but the grasshopper did not." (Female, age 8, Middle Eastern)

These three narratives, then, depict the learning of three different values—not to be wasteful, to be helpful to others, and to have a sense of responsibility. Indeed, classic moral stories are used extensively to teach children about consequences of good and bad behavior (Henderson & May, 2005). Legends, formal storytelling, religious books, often-repeated stories, and children's storybooks (which have the advantage of being written in the children's zone of proximal development) are all vehicles for teaching positive social behavior. Storytelling has, however, received only modest amounts of attention from developmental psychologists, in spite of the fact that parents discuss emotion- and value-related lessons more frequently while reading picture books than they do in everyday conversations (Sabbagh & Callanan, 1998).

Studies that have looked at the effects of storytelling have addressed several issues. One has to do with what kinds of content are more likely to have an effect on children's positive behavior. K. Lee et al. (2014), for example, compared the impact of three often-told stories with a moral theme—"George Washington and the Cherry Tree," "Pinocchio," and "The Boy Who Cried Wolf"—with that of a control story, "The Tortoise and the Hare." In their study, children were first left alone, having been told not to look at or play with an attractive toy the researcher left in the room. A substantial proportion of the children, in fact, disobeyed the researcher and peeked at the toy. When the researcher returned, children were read one of the four stories and then were asked if they had looked at or touched the forbidden toy. Those who had heard about George Washington were less likely to lie to the researcher than were children in the other three conditions. Lee et al. suggest that this was because the Pinocchio and wolf stories focus on the negative consequences of antisocial behavior: Pinocchio's nose grows longer whenever he tells a lie, and when a wolf does appear in the wolf story, no one believes the boy, and the wolf eats his sheep. In contrast, when George Washington tells the truth about chopping down the cherry tree, his father focuses on the positive, praising him for his honesty. When Lee and his colleagues rewrote the George Washington story so that it focused on the negative consequences of dishonesty, the amount of lying increased to the same level as for the other stories. In a later study, Talwar, Yachison, and Leduc (2016) evaluated children's willingness to lie when asked to do so by an adult who had accidentally broken a toy the adult had been told not to touch. Children who heard the George Washington story (in its original form) were more likely to tell the truth than those who heard "The Boy Who Cried Wolf" or "The Tortoise and the Hare."

Other studies have focused on adult–child discussions of emotion in stories and ways in which these discussions can be used to change the child's behavior. In an intervention study (Grazanni, Ornaghi, Agliati, & Brazzelli, 2016), for example, teachers were trained to tell stories to toddlers. The main characters in the stories were two rabbits who, in the course of a series of adventures, felt scared, happy, angry, or sad, and who solved their problems by engaging in some form of prosocial behavior. Teachers used the story content to talk about emotions (in particular, their expression, causes, and regulation), as well as prosocial behavior (such as helping and comforting others). Children were encouraged to talk about when they or others had experienced the emotion under discussion. Compared to a control group, those in the intervention group showed increases in talk about mental states and in prosocial behavior toward their peers.

Studies that include mothers and their toddlers have also demonstrated the important role that stories can play in children's social development. In one study, mothers and children were observed while reading a wordless picture book about a family going on a picnic. The pictures were of family members looking happy, sad, angry, fearful, surprised, disgusted, guilty, and excited. The investigators found that the more mothers talked about positive emotions during their storytelling, the less likely their children were to attribute anger incorrectly to another person, and the less likely they were to be physically aggressive with their peers (Garner, Dunsmore, & Southan-Gerrow, 2008). In another study of very young children and storytelling, Brownell, Svetlova, Anderson, Nichols, and Drummond (2013) observed parents (mostly mothers) reading age-appropriate books to their toddlers. Toddlers who were asked by their parents to label and explain emotions in the stories were subsequently seen to help and share more quickly, especially in the case of prosocial tasks that required more complex emotion understanding. Importantly, it was parents' eliciting of children's talk about emotions, rather than the parents' own production of emotion labels and explanations, that related to prosocial behavior. Once again, this finding underlines the importance of scaffolding in socialization.

## Talking and Socialization of Values

Stories provide a good jumping-off point for discussions about positive social behavior. But caregivers also talk about values and standards in the abstract, without a story around which to frame the discussion. Here are some narratives describing a time when a parent and child talked about values, either because the child asked a question that began a dialogue about a particular value, or because the parent decided it was time to talk about a particular issue. The first three begin with the child's questioning some aspect of the misfortune of others, and the last with a parent's decision to talk about an important value—being persistent and tough.

"After a huge earthquake in Bam, Iran my mom and I were watching the news. I was devastated to see the kind of suffering that took place as a result of the disaster. I complained to my mom, telling her I wished there was something I could do. I told her that living so far away, and being so young, there was no way I could make a real, lasting difference in the lives of the victims. My mom told me I was wrong, and that I COULD make a difference, even if small, it would be just as valid. I sat brainstorming with her for a few hours and decided to do a fund raising event at my elementary school. For Valentine's day, myself, my mom and several friends and family made small Hershey's kisses packaged to be sold for 50 cents. Every lunch hour and recess, I would sell the packages and eventually raised over $500. I made a check out to the Red Cross and was very proud of my accomplishment." (Female, age 7, Middle Eastern)

"There was a debate in my history class about whether the First Nations where robbed of their lands by Europeans. Many of the arguments presented by the students were baseless and included comments that implied that the First Nations were a backwards people, and it was a matter of time before they were conquered, and how the First Nations were a lazy group of people who do nothing but booze and do drugs (where they pointed out current statistics of First Nation youth on reserves). I did not at all agree with this argument, but my main reason for disagreeing was based on rational, logical arguments and what had occurred in history. Again, when I talked to my father about this, he was concerned at my lack of emotion concerning this (and many other issues like this), and somewhere along the line he taught me the importance of empathy. It was a very shocking experience for me to have the male in my household teach me to 'feel' for other people. Most males in the culture I grew up in try to be macho and want to be rational because they think being emotional is a female attribute. To have my father tell me that I should be in touch with my emotional side, and that emotions aren't a hindrance but rather they enhance my experience with other people was a huge learning in itself, but also I learnt a great deal about what kind of man my father was." (Male, age 15, South Asian)

"I was in my community church and the priest told the parish that next week there was going to be a share life collection, which is a collection for starving third world countries when going home after church i asked my father why we had to give our money away to other people. that if we gave our money away I couldn't get all the toys that i wanted. he then told me a story from when he was a little boy in a little village near Lyon. he told me that he had 7 other brothers and sisters and that come dinner time he would have a tiny piece of bread with the smallest piece of meat that you can possibly imagine. he told me but it was enough so that nobody starved. now that his situation is not the same that he is older and that he has more than enough food and money, he told me that you must not forget about other people. they still go through those hardships everyday. just because we are not in those predicaments, we should turn a blind eye to others. we must help them, so that they do not starve or go through unnecessary hardships. the next week i was more than happy to put money in the collection basket." (Male, age 10, Western European)

"It was summer time after my high school graduation. I went back to Taiwan to spend time with my family before leaving Vancouver and heading to Toronto. My parents anounced that we were going to have a family meeting, a more formal one unlike talking during dinner. There wasn't a specific topic. During the meeting, my parents shared their struggles while they were young, and how they fought through it to have the success they have right now and build the family that raised us. The conversation converged toward the concept of persistence and being tough which they wanted to share with us. It was one of the most delighted moment of my life because I knew I was going to leave the family and study in Toronto on my own. I wanted to be tough and never let them down. I wanted them to be proud of me." (Male, age 18, East Asian)

Children's questions and comments about various issues begin at an early age. They include conversations about occurrences in the past, feelings and thoughts in the present, and anticipation of the future. In a study of 4-year-olds and the conversations they had with their mothers, Tizard and Hughes (2002) comment on the wide variety of topics that are discussed, including other family members; growing up; birth, illness, and death; and what people do for a living. Dunn and Hughes (2014) note that the content of young children's talk includes moral choice and judgment, justifications for what is allowed and what is not, and questions about what is fair and what is unfair. They report that early conversations about family rules are complex. Children contradict and insist on their own point of view. When they misbehave, they provide reasons for their acts, including justifications and excuses. They assign blame for bad behavior to someone else. Often the conversations are conducted in a teasing fashion, and the disputes are sources (for the children at least) of pleasure and amusement. Their conversations, then, show how, with the help of parents, very young children are developing an increasingly sophisticated understanding of societal rules. In the course of reaching this understanding, they actively question, rebel, challenge, disagree, and negotiate. The notion of help by parents is important, and highlights the significance of co-constructing rules. In conversations that are effective in teaching values, children's actions are scaffolded until internalization occurs. Scaffolding requires an elaborative style on the part of the parents, with the use of clarifying questions and following up of children's comments so that conversation is extended.

An example of scaffolding of conversations comes from a study by O'Neal and Plumert (2014, p. 488). They observed mothers and their 8- to 10-year-old children talking about safety issues. Each mother and child were shown pictures of children engaging in dangerous activities, such as walking up a slide, climbing on top of a roof, reaching for a pot over a hot stove burner, and climbing on the kitchen counter. The discussion began with each member of the dyad being asked to rate how dangerous the situations were. Mothers then encouraged their children to talk about the safety of the activities when there was disagreement in their ratings, but they also guided their children to the mothers' own way of thinking. One conversation, for example, went as follows:

> **Mother:** What about this one?
>
> **Child:** Very safe.
>
> **Mother:** (*Laughs*) I said kind of unsafe (*points to "kind of unsafe" on the rating scale*) because what if she fell? (*Points away from girl toward the ground.*) I mean, she's not up too high yet (*points from girl to top of slide*), but she's headed there.
>
> **Child:** Yeah, and if she (*points to top of slide*).
>
> **Mother:** What if she couldn't reach up there? (*Points to top of slide.*)

**Child:** Then she might fall.

**Mother:** Yeah. Okay. What do you think we should say?

**Child:** Kind of unsafe.

**Mother:** Okay. I agree.

In O'Neal and Plumert's study, mothers encouraged their children to make the first rating, presumably in order to gain a better understanding of their children's thinking. This understanding, then, helped them tailor their message so as to alter their children's thinking to be more in line with their own. Indeed, disagreements were typically resolved in favor of the mothers.

Another way in which parents utilize the guided learning domain to teach is by "pre-arming" their children so they can deal with stressful events. One class of stressful events that has received particular attention is racial discrimination. African American parents teach their children about the possibility of discrimination and how to respond to it (Hughes & Chen, 1997). In the course of this teaching, they alert their children to the presence of competing values and provide them with arguments and strategies that can help them cope. Another way that parents socialize children so they can deal with racial discrimination is by talking about their cultural heritage and history and explaining how to appreciate diversity and cultural differences. This kind of learning has also been shown to attenuate the negative effects of discrimination in both African American and Asian American adolescents (Atkin, Yoo, & Yeh, 2018; Wang & Huguley, 2012).

## Scaffolding and Socialization of Behavior

Scaffolding and working within a child's zone of proximal development are important for teaching that involves conversation about a whole variety of issues, including values and how to deal with unpleasant emotions such as distress and anger. It can also involve teaching that is focused more on the child's behavior. Caregivers engage in guided learning when they try to teach children specific ways of behaving, including how to help, how to share, how to be polite, how to handle social interactions in a skillful way, and so on. As an example, Hammond and Carpendale (2015) observed mothers' scaffolding of their children's involvement in cleaning up after a tea party and assessed how much they included their young children in the task, as well as the age-appropriateness of their efforts. Mothers' actions ranged from doing nearly all the cleaning themselves with no effort to engage their children, or even interfering with their children's efforts, to integrating their children's interest in particular activities (e.g., picking up cups) into the larger cleanup. Not surprisingly, mothers who scaffolded their children's helping behavior had children who were subsequently more helpful.

Is scaffolding children's behavior simply a way of modeling that behavior so children can imitate it? In a large study of a nationally representative sample of American adolescents, Ottoni-Wilhelm, Estell, and Perdue (2014) compared the effects of parents talking to their adolescents about donations and volunteer work; parents modeling of prosocial behavior such as donations to charity and volunteer work; and the broad parenting dimensions of warmth and support, behavioral control, and psychological control. Both conversations and modeling were independently associated with the adolescents' reports of their own prosocial behavior, and these associations were much stronger than those with parenting dimensions. It would seem, then, that guided learning of behavior and modeling of behavior are distinct entities.

SUMMARY▪ ▪ ▪ ▪ ▪ ▪ ▪ ▪ ▪ ▪ ▪ ▪ ▪ ▪ ▪ ▪ ▪ ▪ ▪ ▪ ▪ ▪ ▪ ▪ ▪ ▪ ▪ ▪ ▪ ▪ ▪ ▪ ▪ ▪ ▪

Talking about values is important for successful socialization: for it to work there must be give and take between parent and child. Conversations need to be scaffolded, with parents asking for clarification, reflecting back the child's ideas, and avoiding delivery of information in a way that is perceived as preaching. Some conversations about values have an added feature for socialization; these are conversations pertaining to specific experiences that children themselves have had. Reminiscing about these past experiences, then, is another part of the guided learning domain, to which I now turn.

## ▪ CONVERSATIONS INVOLVING PAST EXPERIENCE: REMINISCENCE

Reminiscing is an important part of our social lives. It begins early in the course of development (frequently mixed with talk about values and social norms in general), occurring as often as five to seven times an hour. At least some of the content of this reliving of past experience is made up of conversations about times when children were well behaved, were not well behaved, or were experiencing positive or negative emotions (Miller, 1994). And these conversations allow parents to guide or scaffold their children's learning about what is appropriate social behavior, as well as how to deal with emotional arousal. They also provide opportunities to talk about why certain behaviors are appropriate or inappropriate, as well as about ways of coping. All this learning is better accomplished—more easily internalized, in the Vygotskian sense—some time after the event under consideration, when high levels of arousal have dissipated in both children and parents, and the parent–child dyads are no longer operating in the control or protection domain. The change in domain allows for a greater focus on the parents' messages.

## Reminiscing: Styles and Outcomes

How reminiscing is conducted affects its outcomes. One style that has received considerable attention involves the extent to which parents elaborate on the content of the discussion (Reese, Haden, & Fivush, 1993). Mothers who have a highly elaborative style use open-ended questions ("who," "what," "why," "where"); add details by extending their children's utterances; and embellish the descriptions of events so that they, with their children, are able to construct a meaningful narrative. Those without an elaborative style, in contrast, use closed questions requiring only a "yes" or "no"; simply repeat questions when their children do not respond; and do not create a strong sense of narrative (Reese & Newcombe, 2007). In many ways, then, an elaborative style and scaffolding have overlapping features.

Children of highly elaborative mothers have more detailed memories of past experiences (Reese & Fivush, 1993), and these detailed memories increase their understanding of the messages being transmitted (Laible & Panfile, 2009). Accordingly, mothers' elaboration when talking about past emotional and moral experiences has been linked to emotional understanding and early conscience development (Laible, 2004, 2011). Laible, Panfile Murphy, and Augustine (2013) found that mothers' elaborative style when their children were 42 months old predicted children's emotional understanding, empathy, and endorsement of themselves as moral 6 months later. And in two studies in which mothers were trained to be elaborative, a link between their training and their children's cognitive and emotional outcomes was established (Reese & Newcombe, 2007; Van Bergen, Salmon, Dadds, & Allen, 2009).

## Cultural Differences in Reminiscence

As with discipline and parenting style, there are cultural differences in the way reminiscence is conducted, and these differences often reflect differences in attitudes with respect to family cohesiveness and interrelatedness (Fivush & Wang, 2005; Miller, Fung, Lin, Chen, & Boldt, 2012). When reminiscing about emotional experiences, Western European mothers ask more elaborative questions and focus more on personal themes and autonomy than do Chinese mothers. The latter are more repetitive and focus more on social themes and interactions with others. Chinese mothers frequently talk about expectations for their children's good behavior, including societal norms and values, and they make moral evaluations and offer advice. Their children are encouraged to take the perspective of others, consider their feelings and intentions, and maintain harmony with them. In contrast, Western European mothers reminisce about children's misdeeds less frequently, and when they do, the talk is frequently light-hearted and focused more on the children as the central characters in the stories. Opinions are expressed indirectly, advice is offered gently, and suggestions are favored over commands. Children are encouraged to articulate their feelings and negative emotions, and these are met with sympathy and understanding.

The difference in approaches of these two cultural groups reflects the Western emphasis on egalitarianism and the development of an autonomous self, in contrast to the Chinese emphasis on authority and the development of a self in relation to others. Differences between Chinese and Western mothers probably are also driven by the latter's concern with protecting their children's self-esteem.

## Narratives, Reminiscing, and Identity Development

Through conversations about past events, children are provided with the material required to form a sense of self-identity or a life narrative (Fivush, 2001; Fivush, Haden, & Reese, 2006; Laible & Panfile, 2009). When conversations focus on a child's moral transgressions and prosocial behavior, for example, the development of a sense of the self as a moral person is facilitated. When they focus on other behaviors, such as achievement, creativity, or bravery, they lead to the development of a sense of self as an achieving, creative, or brave person. Laible and Murphy (2014) suggest that reminiscing may be more effective than talking about abstract issues because it is more intimately related to the child's experiences, and therefore the lessons being taught are more likely to be processed and remembered.

During the course of reminiscence, parents scaffold their children's developing ability to create narratives until the children begin to internalize the skills needed to do it on their own. Adults can (gently) steer conversations to issues they feel need to be addressed—for example, how their children might have handled a difficult situation in a better way. Fivush (2004) suggests that children "own" their experience when their parents seek out and validate their recollections and interpretations, but not when they impose interpretations. This imposition of interpretations resembles the informative discussions, perceived as opinionated lecturing, described by Walker et al. (2000). Fivush uses the term "validated voice" to describe an individual's acknowledgment that there are different perspectives, but that one of those, or an integration of perspectives, has been accepted as the individual's own and has not been imposed by some other individual. This approach mirrors the approach to internalization of values described throughout this book.

## Building on Stories about Parents

Talking about one's own transgressions is challenging, given that people generally want to present themselves in a positive light. Thus formulating stories about the transgressions of others is a helpful way of developing positive social values and behavior. Stories about others are often about parental transgressions, and they become particularly important during adolescence, when a narrative identity integrating many different experiences (including those of parents) begins to develop (Fivush, Bohanek, Robertson, & Duke, 2004). Adolescents know and can easily tell stories about the experiences of their parents (Fivush, Merrill, & Marin, 2014), and adolescents whose intergenerational narratives are more elaborate and coherent report fewer internalizing and externalizing problems (Fivush, Bohanek, & Zaman, 2011).

## Sex Differences in Talking about Past Experiences

Not surprisingly, there are differences in how mothers and fathers talk to their boys and girls, as well as what they talk about, in the guided learning domain. Parents are more elaborative in conversations with daughters than with sons (Reese & Fivush, 1993), and mothers are more elaborative and more inclined to talk about negative emotional experiences than are fathers (Zaman & Fivush, 2013). Chaparro and Grusec (2015) asked parents and adolescents to say how likely they would be to talk to each other about minor transgressions they had committed (e.g., forgetting to return a book borrowed from a friend) or minor distressing events they had experienced (e.g., a friend forgot their birthday). Fathers said they would talk more about transgressions than about distressing experiences, whereas there was no difference for mothers. Mothers said they would talk more about distressing events than did fathers. Both parents said they were more likely to talk about distressing experiences with their daughters than with their sons. And both boys and girls said they were more likely to talk to their mothers than to their fathers about both kinds of events. In essence, then, reminiscence may be more likely to happen with mothers than with fathers, and talking about distressing experiences may be more difficult for males than for females. Recall the narrative from a young adult who was asked to talk about a time when he had learned an important value, and his surprise that his father talked to him about being in touch with his emotional side:

"It was a very shocking experience for me to have the male in my household teach me to 'feel' for other people. Most males in the culture I grew up in try to be macho and want to be rational because they think being emotional is a female attribute. To have my father tell me that I should be in touch with my emotional side, and that emotions aren't a hindrance but rather they enhance my experience with other people was a huge learning in itself, but also I learnt a great deal about what kind of man my father was."

## ■ CONCLUSION

The guided learning domain provides opportunities for socialization to take place in a peaceful context where a parent and child can exchange a set of ideas. There is good evidence that it works best when learning is scaffolded, with the ultimate goal being a shared understanding as the parent's position is internalized or taken over as the child's own. In other words, the child comes to "own" a particular point of view (Fivush, 2004). Reminiscence has a special role to play in the learning of values, because it offers the opportunity for individuals to bring together a number of experiences and to extract from them a sense of personal identity, with this identity continuing to direct subsequent actions. Blasi (2004), for example, notes that moral action is more likely to be consistent with moral thinking when the individual has a sense of moral identity and is thereby driven to act in accord with that identity. Guided learning seems a particularly effective way to acquire an identity and, therefore, a particularly effective way to promote internalization.

## CHAPTER 1 SCENARIOS REVISITED

Box 6.1 contains the two scenarios from Chapter 1 that are provided there as examples of the guided learning domain.

In the first scenario, in which father and daughter pass a homeless man on the street, Dad misses an opportunity in Alternative A to talk about others who are less fortunate when he simply dismisses Tara's question. Alternative B, which focuses on being careful around strangers, is a possible approach, although it leaves no room for teaching and discussion or for being sensitive to people's needs. In Alternative C, Tara's father not only talks about what they are seeing, but also uses it as an opportunity to teach the importance of understanding and caring for others.

In the second scenario, about bedtime stories, Dad uses stories in Alternative A as a way of teaching a lesson—how to stay out of trouble. He would have even greater success were he to talk about or scaffold Jimmy's understanding of how to avoid trouble, rather than just telling him how trouble could have been avoided. In Alternative C, Dad encourages discussion or talk about positive values, and he talks "with" rather than "to" his son—a more effective way of teaching values. Discussing feelings, including those that are negative, is a good way of encouraging positive social behavior, but Dad loses such an opportunity in Alternative B when he avoids discussing negative feelings.

## BOX 6.1. Scenarios from the Guided Learning Domain

*Tara (8 years old) and her father walk by a homeless man lying in a doorway. Tara asks her father why he is lying there.*

A. Dad says he's not really sure.

B. Dad says Tara should be careful when she sees strange men loitering in doorways.

C. Dad explains that the man is probably homeless, and talks with Tara about homeless people and the problems they face.

*Jimmy (5 years old) likes to have his father read him stories at bedtime.*

A. Dad reads stories about people who get into trouble, and then tells Jimmy how they could have avoided the trouble.

B. Dad avoids stories where characters are upset or distressed, because they don't provide good models of appropriate behavior.

C. Dad reads stories about being kind to other people or to animals, and then talks about them with Jimmy.

# CHAPTER 7

# Learning Values in the Group Participation Domain

## Observation and Engagement with Others

Humans have evolved as social creatures with an inherent desire to be part of a group—a wish that stems from the need to rely on others for assistance and for resources. When groups are large, it is important for their members to be able to identify those who belong, so that benefits are not mistakenly provided to members of an out-group. Symbols and behaviors that distinguish different groups become important, as well as the belief that one's own group is not just different but better (Brewer, 1999). Examples of this belief are seen in children's preference for and more positive evaluations of their own group (Dunham, Baron, & Banaji, 2008; Sherif & Sherif, 1953), their perception of themselves as more similar to in-group members (Bennett & Sani, 2008), and their eagerness to participate in family routines and rituals (Spagnola & Fiese, 2007). The desire to be like other group members also reveals itself repeatedly as young children pretend to be adults and to imitate their parents' various activities.

In the group participation domain, children and parents are members of the same in-group, with parents conveying to their children what is appropriate behavior in that group, and therefore the nature of their shared identity. Parents encourage socially acceptable actions through their own actions, taking advantage of their children's desire to be like others in the group. Parents also work to ensure that children not only are exposed to their parents' displays of acceptable action, but are surrounded by other members of the in-group who also display behavior acceptable to that in-group. Parents encourage friendships of which they approve; they try to live in particular neighborhoods where their children are exposed to positive values; and they attempt to control the amount of antisocial behavior to which their children are exposed in the mass media (and, to the extent possible, in social media). They also encourage their children's participation in rituals and routines, as well as in group activities that help to cement ideas about what is acceptable and appropriate action.

In contrast to the guided learning domain, where parents are teachers who carefully scaffold their children's learning, parents in the group participation domain facilitate their children's learning of values simply by how they act. Additionally, there is no conflict or disagreement, given that children are eager and motivated to be similar to other group members. Observation and participation with others are major ways in which children acquire expectations about a wide range of social actions and attitudes—how to dress, where to eat and sleep, how to behave at the table, how to care for others, what political party to favor, whether to be religious or not, and so on. Indeed, this is the primary mode of learning in cultural communities where knowledge acquisition occurs in the course of daily life, as opposed to in a formal school setting; this form of learning is referred to as "learning by observing and pitching in" (Rogoff et al., 2015).

Certainly much learning in the group participation domain is accompanied by discussion, but much of it also occurs alone, often with little thought or evaluation. There is one major drawback to the use of this strategy, of course: Parents not only need to be aware of the negative values and examples of others, but also need to be careful themselves not to perform antisocial actions or actions that are contrary to what they advocate in the control and guided learning domains (see Figure 7.1, which demonstrates this point).

Children learn values and associated behaviors by observing others. Learning of values also occurs when they actually engage together with others in a designated activity. I begin this chapter with a focus on learning that occurs by observing others, and then move to a discussion of participation with others.

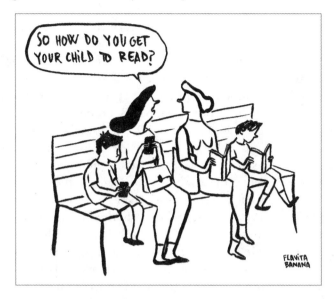

**FIGURE 7.1.** Parenting in the group participation domain: A good and a poor example. Copyright © 2019 by Flavita Banana. Reprinted by permission.

## ■ OBSERVATIONAL LEARNING

Children's learning from watching others has been a topic of considerable interest to developmental psychologists over many years. Sigmund Freud and Robert Sears, for example, spent considerable effort trying to explain how children identify with, or take over, the values of their parents. Neither, however, was able to arrive at a very satisfactory explanation (Grusec, 1992). Sears, for example, in keeping with the perspective of social learning theory that prevailed at the time, attempted to formulate an explanation that involved satisfaction of basic needs as a primary reinforcer; mothers as secondary reinforcers because of their association with primary drive reduction; an acquired dependency motive; and, ultimately, identification with the caregiver. The argument for how this progression might occur, however, was not very convincing. Nor was the Skinnerian argument that new responses could be learned through a process of successive approximation or reinforcement for moving closer and closer to the desired goal. Noting these failures, Bandura and Walters (1963) made the radical suggestion that learning through observation does not depend on reinforcement principles, but is instead a basic form of learning.

A series of experiments carried out by Bandura at Stanford University and Walters at the University of Toronto provided several demonstrations of how children can learn simply by observing the actions of others. Among these were the famous Bobo doll studies (Bandura, Ross, & Ross, 1961, 1963) where children eagerly reproduced the actions of adults who behaved aggressively toward an inflated toy. The results of these studies led to considerable public concern with the effects of violent media (these are discussed later in the chapter). Bandura and Walters also demonstrated that there could be knowledge even in the absence of performance, and that children could be fully aware of the nature and consequences of a given behavior without ever having overtly engaged in it. Thus reinforcement for performing a specific act was unnecessary in order for learning to take place (Bandura, 1977). Similarly, Walters and Parke (1964) found that children did not imitate a model's behavior when it was prohibited, but that they did imitate it when the prohibition was no longer in effect—again an indication that learning could occur without reinforcement. In other studies Bandura and McDonald (1963) questioned the basic tenets of cognitive developmental theorizing about moral development by showing that, through a training procedure involving social reinforcement and modeling, the moral judgments of young children could be modified. And Bandura, Grusec, and Menlove (1967) demonstrated that the anxiety of children who were afraid of dogs could be effectively reduced by having them watch another fearful child exposed to a desensitization procedure. In all, then, observational learning seems a much more efficient technique of behavior change than learning through reinforcement.

Bandura (1977) proposed four steps for successful learning through observation. First, the observer must pay attention to what is being modeled. Variables such as power and attractiveness of the model, as well as how absorbing the presentation is (e.g., television is a compelling medium), affect attention. Next, material must be retained or represented in memory. Then the symbolic representation in memory has to be converted into actions similar to those originally observed. And, finally, there must be sufficient incentive to motivate the actual performance of the actions modeled. The language describing these steps was not that of learning theory, and ultimately it prompted a change in labeling to "social cognitive theory" (Bandura, 1986).

## Learning Values from Observing Others

The following narratives from our young adults illustrate how parents (and occasionally others) influence their children's learning of values simply through modeling behavior related to the value. These narratives include several different values: being helpful, dealing well with adversity, the importance of family, making the most of present opportunities, and remaining positive when things do not go well.

"My dad found a wallet in the mall, and picked it up. Upon coming home, he called the person to whom it belonged and arranged to return it right away, leaving the contents intact and not leafing through their private things." (Male, age 9, Western European)

"When I was in grade 4, my dad made a business deal with someone who wasn't very trustworthy, and it ended up being terminated at the last moment. The man took my dad's money and disappeared. We were just about to move into a new house, which was given as part of the terms of contract in the business deal, so when he disappeared, we were left without a house as well. In the span of two days, my dad had to find a basement for us to stay in temporarily. It was one of the hardest times of my life, because my dad was left without a job, and we didn't have a home of our own. During that time, I took a lot of strength from my mom. The way she reacted to this situation was something I really admired, and I appreciated her strength and acceptance." (Female, age 9, South Asian)

"This event took place when my older brother was accepted into medical school. He was accepted into one of his last choice medical schools but instead of being negative about it and waiting another year to repeat the MCAT [Medical College Admission Test], he took the opportunity. I learned from this event to always be positive and to take different opportunities while you have them and not rely on what 'could have' happened." (Male, age 17, Middle Eastern)

"One night, my father and I were in the car, driving back home from an event. On the way, we saw this lady whose car was stuck in the middle of the road, and she was struggling to remove something from underneath her car. We could have just driven past her car, as there was enough space to do so. Instead, my father stopped our car and went towards the lady's car to help her remove the basket stuck under her car. Within a few minutes, the basket was removed and the lady was able to drive easily." (Female, age 10, South Asian)

"When I was 8 years old my family and I were involved in a car accident that left my mom severly injured. She broke her back and the prognosis was not good; the doctors questioned whether she would ever walk again. However for my mom this was not an option; my mom is a very strong willed and determined person and when she sets her mind to something it gets done. In this case she set her mind to recovery. At such a young age watching someone so influential in your life go through something like that is hard and confusing but I learned a lot from it. I watched my mom progress from being on her back in a hospital bed, to learning to walk again, to walking with a walker, slowly becoming more independant and going to physiotherapy 3 times a week, and aquatherapy 2 times a week to gain back strength. Soon she was walking with a cane and today my mom is able to walk without the use of any aid. There are still some things she cannot do because of her injury, but it's hard to know unless you know her very well. Throughout this whole process my father remained a rock for her, doing whatever she needed to get better while at the same time recognizing that what she wanted help with and what she needed help with sometimes were two different things and challenging her. He was an unequaled support system for her. Both of my parents worked hard to overcome this giant obstacle in an admirable way." (Female, age 8, Western European)

## Observational Learning through the Media: Effects on Children's Antisocial and Prosocial Behavior

Bandura's research on the modeling of aggressive behavior gained widespread attention beginning in the late 1960s—attention that has continued to this day. Much of this attention has been focused on children's learning from aggression that they observe in the mass media. Thus more than a thousand studies have focused on both the short-term and long-term effects of viewing media violence. And a considerable number of meta-analyses have generally confirmed the hypothesis that watching media violence—including aggressive material on television and in the movies, as well as playing violent video games—has long-lasting effects on children's antisocial behavior (Prot et al., 2015).

Studies indicate that children who watch a great deal of violence on television or who play violent video games become desensitized to violence, as well as learning that aggressive behavior is acceptable and enjoyable (Bushman & Huesman, 2010). They also become less empathic and less prosocial (Fraser, Padilla-Walker, Coyne, Nelson, & Stockdale, 2012; Krahé & Möller, 2010). In a study specifically focused on television violence, Huesmann, Moise-Titus, Podolski, and Eron (2003) found that children who viewed more televised violence were more aggressive 15 years later, no matter how aggressive they had been as children. In other words, television violence had a negative impact not just on children who were already attracted to and engaged in antisocial acts, but on all children who witnessed it. In a meta-analysis of studies of violent video games—including experimental, cross-sectional, and longitudinal studies, as well as studies conducted in a variety of Western European countries and in Japan—Anderson et al. (2010) found support for the hypothesis that exposure to violent video games is a causal risk factor for aggressive cognitions (e.g., positive attitudes toward aggression), aggressive affect (anger), and aggressive behavior, as well as decreased empathy and prosocial behavior. They noted that these effects, while statistically significant, were small. Nevertheless, they argued that when large portions of the population are exposed to a risk factor, or when consequences are severe or accumulate across time, small effects become more important (Abelson, 1985). These conditions are all present in the case of violent video game effects.

Although most of the research has focused on aggression, studies have indicated that other undesirable forms of behavior can also be promoted by media exposure. Exposure to alcohol use is related to the early onset of alcohol consumption and binge drinking among adolescents (Wills, Sargent, Gibbons, Gerrard, & Stoolmiller, 2009). Exposure to violent sexual material has been shown to lead to increased sexually aggressive behavior by children and adults (Ybarra, Mitchell, Hamburger, Diener-West, & Leaf, 2011). And a meta-analysis by Oppliger (2007) documented the relation between presentation of gender stereotypes in the media and gender-stereotypic attitudes and behaviors.

Prosocial content in the media has received much less attention than aggressive content. Nevertheless, there are enough studies to enable the assertion that such content has a positive effect on children. Coyne et al. (2018) found that, on the whole, exposure to prosocial media was positively linked to empathy and prosocial behavior, and negatively to aggression. With respect to moderators, they had expected to find that the effects would be stronger for video games and virtual reality, because those require active participation on the viewer's part and thereby provide a more immersive experience. In contrast, television and movies require only passive watching and no demand for constant attention. Coyne et al. found the opposite, however, possibly because prosocial messages may be rarer in video games. Coyne et al. also found that prosocial content assessed in longitudinal studies was associated with prosocial behavior directed toward strangers, but not toward family members and friends. One explanation for this finding is that prosocial behavior toward family is more likely to be motivated by the quality of the relationship, including greater frequency of reciprocity, whereas other motives such as empathy may be more important in behavior toward strangers. Finally, prosocial media had stronger effects on helping and prosocial thinking than they did on donating or volunteering—a reflection of possible differences in amount of portrayal in media of these different forms of prosociality.

Positive effects of media content in other areas have also been demonstrated. For example, music with lyrics emphasizing gender equality leads to more positive attitudes and behavior toward women (Greitemeyer, Hollingdale, & Traut-Mattausch, 2015).

## Protecting Children from the Negative Impact of Media Value Presentations

Given all the evidence that violent television and video games—ubiquitous features of daily life—pose serious problems for the socialization process, what can parents do to minimize their negative impact? It is not always easy to control what children see and do, particularly as they grow older and spend more time away from home, and as their circle of friends and acquaintances widens. How, then, can parents manage situations where their children are viewing or engaging in behavior of which they disapprove?

Goodnow (1997) identified two strategies parents use when their children are confronted with conflicting messages or values. The first is "cocooning"—an approach that protects children from outside influences, although obviously it becomes more difficult to cocoon children as they grow older. The second strategy is "pre-arming" (already mentioned in the discussion of guided learning in Chapter 6), in which children are provided with ways of dealing with values and events that have yet to occur. Added to these two approaches are those of "compromise" and "deference" (Padilla-Walker & Thompson, 2005). Compromise occurs when parents grant some degree of autonomy to their children, while maintaining a degree of control (e.g., limiting contact with the source of conflicting values or messages). Deference occurs when children are allowed to make decisions on their own about degree of exposure; it can happen either in response to a struggle between parent and child, or as part of an active demonstration of the parent's confidence in the child's ability to withstand the negative influence.

In a meta-analysis of various types of strategies parents use when trying to restrict the influence of television, video games, and the internet, Collier et al. (2016) compared "restrictive mediation" and "active mediation" on the effects of viewing aggressive and mature content. Restrictive mediation included cocooning and rule setting, with parents limiting time spent watching TV, playing video games, or on the internet, as well as restricting content including violence and mature subject matter. Active mediation included pre-arming and discussion, with parents attempting to promote critical thinking about media content. Collier et al. also included a comparison of restrictive and active mediation with "co-viewing," where parents either watched with their children because they were concerned about material being viewed, or simply stayed in the same room as the children. They found that restrictive mediation (cocooning) negatively predicted amount of time spent watching TV, as well as sexual behavior such as unwanted early sex, pregnancy, and sex with multiple partners. The first finding—less time spent watching TV—is hardly surprising, but important; as Collier et al. note, it may explain some linkages between time spent with media and child outcomes such as poor academic performance and physical well-being. The second finding—sex-related behavior problems— suggests that cocooning decreases a child's exposure to mature content. Active mediation (pre-arming) predicted later and fewer negative sexual outcomes, as well as reduced aggression and substance abuse. It would appear, then, that discussion about principles and values that are violated in television or video games or on the internet might be one useful way to minimize the negative impact on these values, or even to promote acceptance of more positive values. Finally, co-viewing was significantly related to higher levels of aggression and media use, strongly suggesting that watching television or playing video games with children gives implicit approval for their content, as well as linking such content with pleasant family interaction.

## ■ RITUALS, ROUTINES, AND ENGAGEMENT WITH OTHERS

Group participation includes involvement in rituals and routines, as well as active engagement with others in activities that are relevant to the learning of values. Here are two sample narratives where active participation in positive action promoted the learning of a value.

"When I was 13 years old I began to volunteer in my mom's classroom (she taught an associated class which ranged from children with Autism, developmental delays, down syndrome etc). At first I was very nervous because I had very little experience working with anyone with these types of special needs. My mom was absolutely amazing with these children! And at this moment taught me the value of helping others. She truly wanted to help these children in every aspect of their lives, and the children were extremely responsive to this. I remember thinking that this is what I wanted to do, help others gain what these children had from my mom." (Female, age 13, Western European)

". . . My school rugby team made the final that year, and headmaster decided to take the whole school to Vancouver to support the team. It was a really exciting match. We were screaming and cheering. The team was losing at halftime, but they kept fighting back. We were singing our school hymn during the match to tell the team that we were all behind them. Although we lost the match, we were all proud of the team and ourselves. I learned that teamwork is not only from the team, it is from all the people around you who cares about you." (Male, age 16, East Asian)

## Rituals and Routines

### Rituals

Rituals are symbolic activities that underline group belongingness and thus reinforce the importance of in-group membership. They include a wide variety of events such as national holidays, remembrance days, thanksgiving celebrations, and religious observances. By observing and participating in these rituals, people become more closely bound to each other, and their group-based values are underscored. When rituals are disrupted, family cohesion and group-based values are threatened. Rituals include memorable occasions such as marriages, funerals, graduation ceremonies, coronations, and parades; they function to underline the special nature of one's own social group and the importance of its behavioral requirements.

### Routines

Routines, in contrast to rituals, require a momentary time commitment and, unlike rituals, involve little afterthought once they are completed. When they are disrupted, the disruption is simply a hassle, rather than a serious threat to group solidarity. Nevertheless, routines are important because they can include positive social behaviors performed in ways that are regular and automatic. Thus practices such as getting ready for bed, doing homework at a particular time, dressing in a particular way, or conduct at mealtime all have meaning because they reflect group membership and values, and also because their frequent repetition entrenches them (Davidov, 2013; Fiese et al., 2002; Rossano, 2012; Spagnola & Fiese, 2007).

## HOUSEHOLD CHORES

Household chores are examples of routines that have implications for the development of prosocial values and actions. Staub (1979) suggested that children who perform household chores develop sound work habits, as well as a sense of helping others and being responsible for their welfare. Assisting with household chores also promotes a belief in the self as a helpful person, a sense of agency or personal efficacy, and an appreciation of the needs and feelings of others. Accordingly, these are often the goals of parents who require that their children be helpful in the home, even though it is often easier to perform the work themselves. Indeed, doing work around the house is one of the major sources of family conflict in adolescence (Smetana, 1988), and yet parents continue to persevere in their demands, presumably because they think the effort is a worthwhile one.

Although the argument for positive outcomes with respect to assignment of duties makes sense, the findings in fact have been mixed, with involvement in household work linked to positive social outcomes in some cases but not in others (Goodnow, 1988). A distinction between the way in which work is assigned and the kind of work that is assigned sheds light on some of the confusion. Parents ask children to engage in household work in one of two ways: Either they require that work be done in a routine fashion, or they require it to be done when work or assistance is requested. The former should be a more successful approach, given that engagement in a routine way makes the job one's own and encourages the idea that there is no choice involved. Engagement in response to requests, on the other hand, makes it appear that the task belongs to someone else and therefore does not invoke a sense of responsibility or ownership. Parents can also assign chores of two kinds—either those done for others (such as setting the table for dinner, feeding the dog, and taking out the garbage) or those done for the self (such as making one's bed, doing one's laundry, and cleaning one's room). In this case, doing work that aids others facilitates a concern for the needs of others, whereas doing self-care work does not encourage such a concern.

In a test of these ideas, Grusec, Goodnow, and Cohen (1997) asked mothers and children about the nature and amount of work the children did around the house (fathers were asked as well but were often unsure, as well as being markedly different in their estimates from their children and their wives). Mothers were also asked to keep a journal in which they reported, during prearranged periods of observation, instances in which their children engaged in prosocial behavior by helping others, sharing with them, comforting and defending them, or demonstrating concern for others (including animals as well as people). Grusec et al. found that older children (12–14 years of age) who carried out routine chores that involved work for others were more prosocial. Other combinations of types of chores did not predict prosocial action. Moreover, the same effect was not found for younger children (10–12 years of age)—a suggestion that they had not yet had enough experience with household responsibility for its impact to be reflected on positive behavior. One might argue, of course, that children with a tendency toward helpfulness and cooperation had parents who were more likely to ask for help because compliance would be more likely. This would not explain, however, why the result was confined to one particular form of household work—routines performed for others— and not all forms.

## Engagement with Others

In addition to rituals and routines, group participation includes taking part in activities specifically designed to promote positive social values with other members of the group. These include community service, sports involvement, and after-school activities.

### Community Service

A multitude of opportunities are available for adolescents to engage in community service. In some jurisdictions, such service is actually a requirement for graduation from high school. For example, in the state of Maryland, students are required to complete either 75 hours of student service that includes preparation, action, and reflection, or a locally designed program approved by the State Superintendent of Schools. In the province of Ontario, all high school students must complete 40

hours of community involvement before they can receive their graduation diplomas. Volunteer activity (activity not for pay or credit) is either
recommended or mandated because it allegedly reinforces a sense of
civic responsibility, strengthens the community, enhances the students'
self-confidence and self-image, offers networking for future employment, and provides experiences for students to include in their portfo-
lios (see *www.edu.gov.on.ca/extra/eng/ppm/124a.html*). A broad range of
volunteer activities can satisfy civic service requirements. They include
helping or spending time with seniors, assisting with child care, cleaning up parks, planting trees and flower beds, tutoring younger students,
getting involved with charitable activities or animal welfare agencies,
volunteering in a hospital, and helping at school in the library or with
charitable events. Parents play a role in this requirement, as they often
are asked to provide assistance to their children in selecting community involvement activities, as well as communicating with community
sponsors and the school principal.

Volunteering is an excellent example of group participation—in
this case, getting together with a group to benefit needy individuals or
the environment. It serves many functions that are regarded as beneficial for the development of adolescents' skills and attitudes. Some of the
goals are self-oriented, as they include enhancing self-confidence and
self-image, networking for future employment, and providing material for a resume. But an important goal is teaching young people the
value of helping others. Adolescents learn that they have an obligation
to become aware of social issues, as well as different perspectives, values, and behaviors. They also become sensitive to societal problems,
and, through critical reflection, they see how their actions can have an
impact on others.

In a meta-analysis involving 49 studies, all of which were longitudinal in nature, van Goethem, van Hoof, Orobio de Castro, Van Aken,
and Hart (2014) addressed the effectiveness of community service and
volunteering for achieving its various goals. They were particularly
interested in the role of reflection in promoting these goals. By "reflection," they meant the provision of opportunities in the classroom for
deliberate consideration of volunteer activity. Such consideration
would include contemplation of moral principles, civic obligations,
and social inequalities, along with attempts to connect real-life events
with attitudes and values taught in the classroom. With appropriate
reflection, then, students should be able to use their service to others
as raw material that could form the basis for developing positive values,

attitudes, and social action. van Goethem et al. found that community service yielded moderate positive effects in all areas they assessed: academic content and competence, academic and career attitudes, personal and social competence, attitudes toward the self, attitudes toward others, civic competence, and civic attitudes. The effect was stronger when reflection (specifically, written evaluations, discussion with others, and thinking about the activity by the self) was undertaken more frequently, when the community service was performed more often, and when adolescents were older. Older adolescents were more likely to benefit, presumably because they were better able to integrate their experiences into their self-identities as particular kinds of persons.

Of interest were variables that did not affect the relation between volunteering and outcomes. These included the kind of community service; the extent to which community service involved or did not involve personal contact with vulnerable individuals or groups was not a significant factor in its various outcomes. Boys and girls also did not differ in their responsiveness to community service. And there was no cutoff with respect to amount of service or indication that it might become counterproductive if too much were required: These studies showed a positive effect up to 180 hours. Moreover, it made no difference whether or not the service was required as part of the school curriculum. Although the element of coercion in required service might undermine intrinsic interest or lead to reactance, there was no evidence that this was so in the case of required civic service.

## Sports Involvement

Another form of group participation that has received considerable attention from researchers is involvement in organized youth sports. Findings with respect to the effects of sports participation on various psychosocial outcomes are mixed at best. In their meta-analysis, Evans et al. (2016) point out the complexity of sports activities, which no doubt accounts for these mixed outcomes. These activities vary across sport types, as, for example, in the level of interdependence with teammates; across settings, as in the level of competitiveness involved; and among individual levels of involvement. According to Evans et al., one can conclude overall that youth involvement in sports requiring greater interdependence is associated with enhanced developmental experiences and self-esteem, as well as with lower levels of depression, although very high involvement has been associated with higher levels of depression. However, sports involvement is also associated with lower levels of moral reasoning. It must be noted that even these effects are not consistent across all studies, and that they vary as a function of age and gender.

A significant number of studies have considered the effect of sports involvement specifically on juvenile delinquency. Indeed, in the belief that sport participation is an effective intervention to decrease anti-social behavior, local governments and institutions are keen to offer youth sports activities. The idea is that athletes are too busy to engage in delinquent behavior, or that sports involvement builds character in the form of positive traits, skills, and virtues. It is argued that youth learn to follow rules and standards of behavior, and so acquire virtues such as honesty and fairness; that sports teach youth to deal with set-backs and encourage perseverance and self-control, as well as increasing peer cooperation and acceptance; and that sports lead to greater self-esteem, and therefore less vulnerability to negative peer influences (Spruit, van Vugt, van der Put, van der Stouwe, & Stams, 2016). In opposition to these beliefs, some have argued that the competitiveness of sports can lead to immoral action, such as cheating or injuring an opponent. Excessive alcohol consumption may also be part of the culture of some sports teams (Spruit et al., 2016).

In a meta-analysis that included 132,366 youth, Spruit et al. did not find support for the position that sport participation is either beneficial or harmful with respect to delinquent behavior. They did find some moderators of a relation between sports activities and juvenile delinquency, however, although the results were modest in size. Athletes participating in a school setting were more likely to benefit than those participating in an out-of-school setting. And individual sports were associated with less delinquency, whereas no associations were found for team sports. Although it could be concluded that sports participation has no impact on the delinquent behavior of young people, Spruit et al. propose that a protective influence of sports participation may be attenuated by its negative influences. If this is the case, it means that steps need to be taken to identify the two aspects—protective and negative—and to control them appropriately. For example, the finding that more favorable outcomes were associated with school settings may be explained by the presence of more skilled coaches as opposed to volunteers. As well, in a school setting there are opportunities for consultation between the school and coaches, with subsequent positive results. Team sports promote the practice of social skills and can be beneficial when there is a climate of "fair play" and when the acquisition of skills is considered more important than winning.

In conclusion, then, sports activities may have a positive effect on social development. From what is known so far, the effect may well be stronger for team sports than for individual sports (although the Spruit et al. results were equivocal), and for school-based sports activities.

### After-School Programs

After-school programs constitute another example of interventions that are intended to have positive socialization outcomes through bringing children and adolescents together in a group participation setting. Unlike extracurricular activities that occur after school (including sports or academic clubs), after-school programs offer an array of activities, including play, academic enrichment, community service, sports, and arts and crafts. They are often intended for low-income youth at risk for problems and are provided in settings where cost, availability, and safe travel are of concern to families. These latter types of programs receive significant amounts of financial support from local and national governments, with the intention that they provide a safe haven and supervised time after school, as well as minimizing exposure to deviant models, teaching and promoting new skills, offering opportunities for positive interactions with adults and peers, and curbing juvenile crime. They are alleged to minimize criminal opportunities by influencing the routine activities of participating youth, exposing them to more positive forms of behavior, and reducing unsupervised social interactions through the imposition of structure (Kremer, Maynard, Polanin, Vaughn, & Sarteschi, 2015; Taheri & Welsh, 2016).

In spite of these hoped-for outcomes, meta-analyses of after-school programs by Kremer et al. and by Taheri and Welsh suggest that, overall, they have very little effect on child and adolescent outcomes. The reviewers do not argue that such programs should be discontinued; there is no evidence that they are harmful, and they do provide much-needed services to families. With respect to targets such as the reduction of externalizing behaviors, however, more careful implementation and evaluation of such programs are needed.

### ■ CONCLUSION

Observation and participation have many advantages with respect to the learning of values and of behaviors associated with those values.

They do not occur in the context of emotional arousal and distraction on the part of children, and so attention to messages being transmitted is more easily maintained. Routines that happen in this domain and that involve positive social behavior become automatic, involving continued repetition with little thought. And values acquired in this domain may be particularly well internalized, because they require that children engage in mental effort to extract the messages being conveyed.

Some findings from the narratives collected in my lab suggest additional positive features of the group participation domain (Vinik et al., 2013; Vinik, 2013). We found that prosocial values such as helping others most frequently characterized narratives in the group participation domain, in contrast to narratives from the control domain, where not harming others was most frequently cited as the value learned. This finding no doubt reflects the fact that parents rarely punish failures to be prosocial (Grusec, 1991; Grusec et al., 1982), and it points to the importance of example in the development of concern for others. Next, we found that narratives involving values learned through observation appear to be more coherent or richer in content and to make more sense than those in either the control or the guided learning domain, suggesting that the absence of input by others can require considerable cognitive effort on the part of children to extract the value. This effort results in greater comprehension and remembering and, quite possibly, greater internalization. Finally, we found in narratives in the observational learning domain that the self was cited as the source of value learning more frequently than in any other domain. This finding suggests that values acquired in the observational learning domain could be more likely to be "owned" (to borrow the term from Fivush, 2004), or internalized, than those from the other two domains.

Observation and participation also have their disadvantages. They require effort on the part of parents not to model behavior contrary to what they wish to teach their children (see Figure 7.1). The great many models of antisocial behavior in children's environments require that parents protect or inoculate their children against those models. Nevertheless, learning from watching others and from interacting with others is a ubiquitous feature of everyday life and a powerful means of encouraging children to adopt socially acceptable behavior.

## CHAPTER 1 SCENARIOS REVISITED

Box 7.1 contains the two vignettes that have been provided as examples of the group participation domain in Chapter 1.

In the first example, Terry's parents feel the need to teach their son to be considerate of others. The best response is no doubt Alternative B—caring for animals in the shelter along with his parents. It will be even more useful if there are discussions and reflections about the animals and their needs. Alternative A, keeping Terry from befriending antisocial children, may be useful—although it does not teach him positive behavior, and Terry is also getting old enough to seek out his own friends. Alternative C, playing video games with a prosocial theme, is also a good response, although such games may be more difficult to find than are games with antisocial themes.

In the case of Grace, who wants to watch TV with her mother, Alternative A is a useful one. Although it is somewhat directive, Grace's mother makes her proposal that they watch a program with positive content as a suggestion, and does focus on a movie that has received good reviews. Alternatives B and C do not ensure that the most acceptable program will be chosen, although having a discussion gives Grace's mother a chance to guide Grace toward what her mother considers an acceptable choice.

---

**BOX 7.1.** Scenarios from the Group Participation Domain

*Terry (12 years old) is not as kind and considerate as his parents would like him to be.*

A. His parents make sure Terry does not befriend other children who are antisocial.

B. Terry and his parents routinely visit an animal shelter where they spend time walking the dogs, which Terry enjoys.

C. His parents look for video games Terry can play that have a prosocial theme.

*Grace (8 years old) wants to watch TV with her mother.*

A. Mom suggests they watch a well-reviewed movie about a young woman with a disability who trains hard and wins a medal at the Paralympics.

B. Mom lets Grace choose what program they should watch.

C. Mom and Grace have a discussion about what would be a good program to watch.

# CHAPTER 8

# Final Thoughts

I n this last chapter, I conclude and summarize my discussion of socialization. First, I note that the five domains I have described in this book do not necessarily function in isolation. I then move to significant differences in usage of the domains by mothers and fathers, as well as by different cultural groups. Finally, I talk about features of the control, guided learning, and group participation domains that distinguish them from each other, particularly as they relate to internalization.

## ■ CO-OCCURRENCE OF DOMAINS

Although I have dealt to this point with one domain at a time, the domains often occur together or in close proximity. Consider, for example, the fact that parents not only comfort and alleviate the distress of their children, but also teach them how to deal with distress in an optimal way. They may even model soothing behavior, which the children can then translate into self-soothing actions. In this case, a parent–child dyad is operating in the protection, guided learning, and group participation domains nearly simultaneously. Interactions can also move in quick succession from one domain to another. Thus a temper tantrum might be followed by a need for comfort. In this situation, responses to the temper tantrum need to be modified somewhat, given entry into the new domain. The parent, for example, might acknowledge the need for comfort but also talk about how to deal with frustration in a more appropriate way. Sometimes a value learned in one domain may be different from that learned in another domain. The best example of this, no doubt, is when a parent says one thing in the guided learning domain and does something else in the group participation domain. Consider the mother who is faced with the task of disciplining her child for hitting a sibling and who says, "We don't do that in this house," at the same time as she spanks her child. Or consider a father who talks about the importance of healthy eating habits at the same time as he savors candy and ice cream. Finally, some situations may require that two domains be involved in order to achieve behavior change. Recall from Chapter 7, for example, that the positive effects of community service occur when students have the opportunity to reflect on moral principles, civil obligations, and social inequalities, and to link them to experiences they have actually had in their volunteering activities (van Goethem et al., 2014).

Here are some narratives from our young adults that describe interactions involving more than one domain.

"I was at home with my parents and my cousin's parents. My uncle, had just found out that my cousin had lied to him where she had been and what she was doing. It was a harsh situation. My cousin had said she was at school decorating the gym for a dance, when in fact she had gone to her friend's house to smoke. I was shocked and her parents were furious. My parents were there to support my uncle and I couldn't speak on my cousin's behalf. Later on my parents talked to me about how a child's freedom is built upon credit. If you lie to your parents you lose your credit and your parents can't trust you or respect you anymore. No longer are you free. This lesson helped me to learn to always be truthful to my parents." (Female, age 15, Western European)

In this first narrative, both the group participation and the guided learning domains were activated. The narrator recalls observing the consequences her cousin experiences for lying, and the narrator's parents took advantage of the opportunity to talk about the importance of telling the truth to your parents.

"In high school there was this chemistry test. It was really really hard and most of the class failed it including one of my friends that was always the best student in chemistry. I however, some how got lucky and scored quite high on the exam. I of course was very happy since chemistry was never really my thing and teased my chemistry expert friend previously mentioned about it.

He got mad and went to my back to the teacher and told the teacher i was cheating. The chem teacher summoned me to his office and with some time it was proven that there was no evidence except for the fact that i, being a usual C+ chem student got an A on a test where A students failed it. So there wasnt any actual evidence that i cheated. I was very very angry and confused at my friend. We werent best pals but we ok friends who would say hello everyday and share a light conversation. So being very angry i got my best friend after school and tried to corner the guy who falsely accused me. We did not succeed since he actually went home earlier that day. I went home and told this event to my mother. She told me that physical abuse is not the answer and that just stay away from the kind of person who does this. I need to go talk to him and make it clear that this kind of action will not be tolerated and that if he still wants to be friend then events like this cannot occur again. And also do not try to cause him back any damage, just forgive him for it and do not try to copy his actions in the future. And this is what i do now, treat people around you with a forgiving attitude, and confront them with any thing that they might have done to negatively affect me in anyway. And not try to copy them and do the same thing to them." (Male, age 16, East Asian)

In this narrative, our young adult recalls being angry and upset when falsely accused (protection domain), trying to hurt the accuser (control domain), and learning from his mother how to be forgiving (guided learning domain).

"When I came to Toronto for high school, I came here alone. My parents were back in Hong Kong, I had to face a lot of difficult decisions and went through tough times. My father told me that I have to learn to be independent and solve my own problems as he cannot always be by my side forever. I learned how to be independent and be strong as I will not be able to go back to Hong Kong and had to stay here until I finish University. This molded me into a very independent person, and also brought me to church and found a place that I can share my happiness and sadness. It gave me an opportunity to build religious values." (Female, age 15, East Asian)

Here the young woman was distressed (in the protection domain), and her father showed her that she had to be independent (guided learning domain).

"... I visited India. ... On this occasion I became very aware of the devastating levels and amount of poverty in India. My mother took me to visit a slum in Mumbai and I was shocked by how poor people were. ... After witnessing not only how extreme poverty could be, but also how widespread it was, I talked things over with my mother. . . . She relayed to me that deep poverty was widely prevalent across the world, and told me how privileged I was to have grown up in a middle class household in Canada. The values she taught me were to always be grateful for what I have, to never judge people for their own material conditions, and that the goal of those like me with relative privilege should be to expand the prosperity I am so lucky to experience to the rest of the world." (Male, age 11, South Asian)

Here the young boy was distressed by the poverty he saw (protection domain), and his mother taught him that he should help others to have some of the same privileges he enjoyed (guided learning domain).

## ■ DIFFERENCES BETWEEN MOTHERS AND FATHERS AND AMONG CULTURAL GROUPS

Most of our knowledge about socialization comes from studies of mothers and children in a Western European cultural context. One obvious question is whether there is a difference between mothers and fathers in how they function in, or are comfortable with, different socialization domains. A second question is whether there are differences in domain usage in different cultural contexts.

### Mothers, Fathers, and Domains

Here I summarize some of the differences between mothers and fathers in their actions and effects in various domains; most of these differences have already been discussed in previous chapters of this book. Of course, generalizations about the parenting practices of fathers and mothers will continue to change over time with the changing role of fathers in childrearing, as well as evolving expectations with respect to fathers' appropriate participation in the parenting process.

Hoffman (1970b) argued that power-assertive interventions in isolation are ineffective in changing children's antisocial behavior, and even harmful. He contended that they need to be replaced or modified with the addition of other-oriented reasoning—reasoning that emphasizes the negative impact of misbehavior on others. This is a position that continues to influence thinking about socialization to this day. However, Hoffman also noted that the positive effects of other-oriented reasoning seem to occur only in the case of mothers. Indeed, a number of studies suggest that mothers and fathers have different disciplinary styles. Mothers use more explanations during discipline, and they are more likely to mediate between participants in a conflict and to gather information than are fathers, who are more oriented to ending the interaction. Fathers are more likely to adopt an authoritarian style, characterized by statements such as "I don't want to listen to this. You two button it," or "Don't argue with your mother, you're going" (Vuchinich et al., 1988). Children appear to recognize this difference when they suggest that fathers use more power assertion than do mothers, and moreover that it is acceptable and appropriate for fathers to do so (Dadds et al., 1990; Siegal & Barclay, 1985). Presumably, because children believe that power assertion is acceptable and appropriate when used by fathers but not by mothers, power assertion should be less negative in its impact for fathers than it is for mothers.

Greater assertiveness on the part of fathers also appears when they are seen playing with their toddlers. Lindsey et al. (2010b) observed that fathers were more likely than mothers to lead the play interaction, make polite commands, issue orders, and ignore or reject their children's requests. Mothers, in contrast, were more likely to give their toddlers opportunities to lead the play and more likely to comply with their children's initiations during play. It should be noted that these differences did not occur in a caregiving situation where mothers and fathers were asked to share a snack with their children and where their approaches to the task were similar.

Differences between mothers and fathers in the protection domain have also been noted. Chaparro and Grusec (2015), for example, asked mothers and fathers how likely they would be to talk to their adolescents about mildly distressing events, such as being worried about having to give a presentation. Mothers were significantly more likely to say that they would talk about such events than were fathers. Fathers, on the other hand, did not differ from mothers in how likely they said they would be to talk about minor violations of rules (e.g., being stopped for speeding). Fathers' reluctance to talk about emotion was also evident in the guided learning domain, with mothers more elaborative in their conversational style as well as more inclined to talk about negative emotional experiences (Zaman & Fivush, 2013).

In sum, then, fathers appear to be more power-assertive in the control domain. They are less responsive in the reciprocity/play domain. And they are less willing than mothers to talk about distressing events in the protection and guided learning domains. These differences do not mean that mothers are more effective at facilitating children's value learning than are fathers. It does suggest that expectations with respect to what is normal or usual behavior are important in determining the impact of that behavior on a child. Note that violation of expectations is not always a problem, however. Recall from Chapter 6 the young adult who wrote about a conversation with his father in which his father urged him to be in touch with his emotional side. In this case, the fact that his father's behavior was not normative had a positive effect on his value learning.

## Culture and Domains

Cultural differences in domain-related behavior also occur, although with the world's increasing level of interconnectedness, many of these differences are becoming blurred. As discussed in Chapter 5, the use and the effects of authoritarian parenting styles across cultures have received considerable attention. Authoritarian parenting generally is seen in a more positive light in many settings outside Western European ones, where it is viewed as a sign of caring. In Western European settings, it is more likely to be interpreted in a negative way, particularly given that it is more likely to be associated with a parent's rejection and loss of control. Again, as with differences between mothers and fathers, the meaning assigned to a parenting intervention determines its impact. Although there is no way in which some forms of parenting could be interpreted as benign and well intentioned, there is a continuum that allows for a more or less positive interpretation.

Moving away from the control domain, Rogoff and her colleagues (e.g., Rogoff et al., 2015) have described distinctions among cultures in the use of different learning strategies. They identify three routine cultural practices that organize children's learning in different ways. These are "learning by observing and pitching in," "assembly-line instruction," and "guided repetition of text." Learning by observing and pitching in entails watching what others do, with the intention of joining in that behavior when the rudiments of it have been learned. Thus it seems similar to learning in the group participation domain. Assembly-line instruction occurs when teaching is undertaken by experts, so children can learn the practices of their community without actual involvement of a productive kind. This approach seems to parallel that of the guided learning domain. Finally, guided repetition of text entails a child's observing a model, imitating that model, rehearsing the model's behavior until the skill or task has been mastered, and then performing the behavior so that mastery can be assessed by an expert. Throughout, the expert supervises the novice and may assist, evaluate, or correct as needed, until mastery is achieved. This latter form of learning does not really seem to correspond to any socialization domain, although it is used in all cultures to teach music, athletics, and crafts. Guided repetition of text is most frequently associated with the learning of religious texts, although it has also been identified as a prominent feature of East Asian educational practice. Learning by observing and pitching in is more frequently observed in cultural communities where there is no formal schooling, and assembly-line instruction, of course, is more prominent in Western cultures, both at school and in the home. Guided repetition of text is disparaged by Western teachers and researchers—a possible explanation for why there is not much research evaluating its effectiveness.

## ■ VALUE LEARNING IN THE GUIDED LEARNING AND GROUP PARTICIPATION DOMAINS: SOME COMPARISONS

Analyses of socialization, as well as of childrearing advice, tend to focus heavily on two dimensions of parenting: the nature of the support relationship between parent and child, and the kind of control strategies the parent uses in order to gain compliance (Maccoby & Martin, 1983). I have dealt with support (protection and reciprocity) in Chapters 3 and 4, and with control in Chapter 5. Support includes responsiveness to the child's emotional needs as in the protection domain, as well as the acceptance, responsiveness, and warmth that reveal themselves in the reciprocity domain. Control has to do with the setting of rules, form of discipline, and nature of reasoning that accompanies the discipline. A domains-of-socialization approach offers at least two additional paths to socialization in the form of guided learning and group participation.

One feature that sets these two paths or domains apart from support and control is that they require a parent to take initiative to put them into practice, even when there is no immediate reason to do so. A child's distress, reasonable requests, and misdeeds are compelling with respect to the need for a response. Thus a child who is hurt or afraid demands some response, whether it be comfort or dismissal. A child who asks a parent for a favor must either be granted that favor or refused. A child's bad behavior demands some reaction if one is to be considered a responsible parent. On the other hand, reading storybooks, using a real–life opportunity that arises as a jumping-off point for a discussion about some issue, or monitoring one's own behavior for possible antisocial features all require effort, because they necessitate taking action that is not compelled by the immediate situation. Additionally, however, they provide opportunities for more positive and pleasurable interactions than are afforded by disciplining a child. In sum, then, I am suggesting that guided learning and group participation take effort to implement, but that the payoff for their use is considerable: They provide pleasanter ways of teaching values than discipline, because they reduce the incidence of affectively negative interactions between parent and child. Moreover, their use may reduce the need for interactions in the control domain if potential problems can be anticipated and prepared for.

## ■ INTERNALIZATION VISITED ONCE AGAIN

This book has focused on the central question for socialization theory—how values are internalized so that they continue to influence behavior independently of external conditions. How internalization is proposed to work differs, however, depending on the domain under consideration.

### Internalization in the Control and Guided Learning Domains

That the conceptualization of internalization in the control and guided learning domains differs is not surprising, of course, given that control and guided learning have emerged from quite different theoretical traditions. To summarize the research findings presented in Chapter 5, internalization in the control domain refers to individuals' beliefs that they have behaved in accord with a given value because that belief is self-generated. When asked why they would help another person, those who have successfully internalized a prosocial value would say it was because it was the proper and appropriate thing to do. They would not say that they were helpful because someone would approve if they helped (or disapprove if they didn't help), or because they would feel guilty if they didn't help, or because the person they helped was expected to return the favor. Similarly, people who have internalized the value of honesty and respect for others do not behave in a positive way to avoid going to jail. They do so because they believe that equality, respect, and fairness are important principles guiding human interaction. Parenting strategies that promote internalization include mild levels of power assertion, along with reasoning that makes sense in response to the misdeed, that is understood correctly, and that focuses on the harm done to others. Under these conditions, values are internalized because a child's feelings of choice or autonomy have not been undermined.

Contrast this depiction of internalization with that in the guided learning domain. Here, as detailed in Chapter 6, the emphasis is on careful attention to the way in which discussions about values are addressed, in order for children to achieve complete understanding of what those values are. In this domain, internalization is a process whereby parents (and other teachers) work within the confines of children's current understanding, but provide temporary support for reaching higher levels of comprehension. Supportive strategies in the form of scaffolding are removed when they are no longer needed; when this happens, children are seen to have taken over the teachers' position and made it their own. Not only do they accurately perceive their teachers' value, but they have also been encouraged, through a process of give and take, to take ownership of it—that is, to accept it as their own. Parent–child dialogue in this domain requires cooperation and collaboration between teacher and student. It requires reflection and restating of the other person's position. The provision of information in a didactic way is not successful, because it is too much like preaching. In other words, didactic teaching undermines feelings of autonomy. And what an analysis in terms of scaffolding does is to show in specific detail how a student's feelings of autonomy can be supported.

### Autonomy Support in Parent–Child Conversations

Consider the following two scenarios. In both, mother and child have witnessed an incident involving two unfamiliar children on the playground: A girl dumped a bucket of sand on her brother's head, he retaliated by pinching her, and the girl started to cry. The mother sees this as an excellent opportunity to teach her child about how problems can be handled without resorting to aggressive action. The first scenario depicts an approach that could be described as autonomy-supportive or well scaffolded, as the mother asks leading questions and reflects on her child's answers. The second scenario is highly directive and offers little opportunity for the child to reflect or react.

### SCENARIO 1

**Child:** Look, Mom! He pinched her!

**Mother:** Oh, dear! Well, here comes the babysitter to solve things.

**Child:** Someone's going to get in trouble.

**Mother:** Well, honey, who do you think should get in trouble?

**Child:** The girl threw sand at him first. That's mean! She started it!

**Mother:** But isn't pinching mean, too?

**Child:** Yeah, I guess so, but I think it's okay since the girl started it.

**Mother:** (*Pause*) Hmmm. Do you really think being just as mean makes things better?

**Child:** Yeah.

**Mother:** Yeah? (*Pause*) How?

**Child:** It made him feel better.

**Mother:** Maybe at that time, but (*pause*) how will he feel later?

**Child:** I think he will feel bad about it later when he gets into trouble.

**Mother:** That could be right. And now that the girl is crying, he can see that he really hurt her! So what else besides pinching do you think he could do to fix the problem?

**Child:** Tell her he didn't like it, and not to do it again?

**Mother:** That sounds like a good idea. Also, who else could he talk to?

**Child:** The babysitter?

**Mother:** How would talking to the babysitter help?

**Child:** That way the girl won't get hurt, and he won't get into trouble.

### SCENARIO 2

**Child:** Look, Mom! He pinched her!

**Mother:** Oh, dear! Well, here comes the babysitter to solve things.

**Child:** Someone's going to get in trouble.

**Mother:** *Both* of them should get into trouble!

**Child:** Why? She threw sand at him first. That's mean.

**Mother:** Pinching is mean, too. *Both* should get into trouble, because people should get into trouble for doing mean things. You should never be mean to people, no matter what. Just because someone is mean to you, you can't be mean back.

**Child:** But she started it! She threw sand at him!

**Mother:** There are a lot of other ways to solve the problem. Talking to your mother or the babysitter, talking to the girl who threw sand, asking her not to do it, moving away, playing somewhere else. . . . Pinching is wrong!

### Reminiscence

Reminiscence in the guided learning domain may well have a singularly important role to play in internalization. As I have noted in Chapter 6, reminiscing about past experiences provides material for the development of a self-identity. When discussing past examples of their own positive and negative actions, children come to think of themselves as exemplars of particular characteristics—morality, kindness, ambition, creativity—and these self-identities guide their behavior so that it is consistent with those characteristics. Thus they have not only internalized a single value, but have developed an identity that includes many exemplars of that value.

## Internalization in the Group Participation Domain

A distinctive feature of the group participation domain is that the observer needs to infer the nature of the value being displayed. Vinik et al. (2013), when they asked young adults to describe a time they had learned an important value, also asked them from whom they had learned the value. Most frequently cited as the source of values were parents, peers, the self, and authority figures such as teachers. In the group participation domain, the greater proportion (approximately two-thirds) of the values learned were attributed to the self—a substantially greater percentage than occurred in the other domains. Presumably, in the group participation domain, agents of socialization are not present to assist in learning a value through reasoning or discussion. The value has to be inferred by the self; this is a perfect way, of course, for internalization to take place. The following narrative from the group participation domain is a good example of how individuals have to do the work of extracting a value by themselves.

> "On Sunday I volunteer at a hospital, where I deal with in-patients who are recovering form surgery. Most of the patients are elderly, but there is this one elderly women that left an impression on me. She was 99 years old and she was so positive about the world and thankful for life, which is very different from most of the other elderly patients we see. I have seen many of the patients start to cry because they think they are useless and that there is no reason left for them to live. This positive elderly woman taught me to appreciate life and my family. I now spend more time with my family and make more of an effort to be pleasant to them and not to take out my stress on them."
> (Female, age 14, Western European)

## SUMMARY ■ ■ ■ ■ ■ ■ ■ ■ ■ ■ ■ ■ ■ ■ ■ ■ ■ ■ ■ ■ ■ ■ ■ ■ ■ ■ ■ ■ ■ ■ ■ ■ ■ ■ ■ ■

I have suggested that internalization of values can be achieved in several different ways, depending on the particular domain of socialization that is activated. The first is through the use of moderate and appropriate levels of power assertion, accompanied by appropriate reasoning; in this way, behavior associated with the value is seen to be inherently correct, rather than motivated by fear of punishment or feelings of guilt. The second is through scaffolding of levels of comprehension until the value is taken over or owned. And finally, the value can be deduced by the observer so that it is seen as self-generated.

## ■ DOMAINS AS A USEFUL FRAMEWORK FOR UNDERSTANDING SOCIALIZATION: A FINAL LOOK

Much of the confusion that arises when parents are provided with conflicting advice about teaching values to their children, or when students and researchers are presented with a set of findings that do not always appear to hang together, can be solved by understanding that socialization occurs in many different ways. These different ways have been the topic of this book.

To recap, in the protection domain, children learn that they can trust their parents to protect them when they are in danger; in the reciprocity domain, they experience positive exchanges with their parents that make for willing compliance with parental directives. Success in these two domains creates a positive relationship that underlies and contributes to success in the other three domains, which involve specific teaching of values. In the control domain, this teaching consists of attempts to modify or improve behavior by applying consequences and explanations for why a certain behavior is correct and another behavior is wrong. This is the domain where the nature of the parent–child relationship may be particularly important, given that consequences and explanations have different meanings, depending on whether they are applied in a context of caring/acceptance or of hostility/rejection. The control domain is frequently associated with anger, frustration, distress, and even shame on the part of parents, with these emotions threatening to derail appropriate parenting strategies. The last two domains, guided learning and group participation, both occur in a more positive context and can be excellent venues for internalizing or taking over of values as inherently correct and self-generated.

Across the control, guided learning, and group participation domains, one principle that frequently emerges is the importance of supporting a child's feelings of autonomy. Control must be applied in a way that is not coercive, but encourages the child to feel that values are inherently correct and self-chosen. Discipline must not be excessive, and reasons must make sense. Teaching discussions must be conducted so that the exchange includes a consideration of both points of view, rather than the imposition of the parent's view on the child. Group participation must not feel forced or pressured. A second principle has to do with perceptions of parent intent. A belief that parental intentions are positive and emerge from caring, acceptance, and responsiveness are central aspects of the socialization process. When these two conditions are present—autonomy support and a positive perception of parental action—the stage is set for the successful preparation of children to live positive and fulfilled lives in a socially responsible way.

# References

Abelson, R. P. (1985). A variance explanation paradox: When a little is a lot. *Psychological Bulletin, 97*, 129–133.

Ainsworth, M. D. S., & Bell, S. M. (1970). Attachment, exploration, and separation: Illustrated by the behavior of one-year-olds in a strange situation. *Child Development, 41*, 49–67.

Ainsworth, M. D. S., Blehar, M. C., Waters, E., & Wall, S. (1978). *Patterns of attachment: A psychological study of the Strange Situation*. Hillsdale, NJ: Erlbaum.

Aksan, N., Kochanska, G., & Ortmann, M. R. (2006). Mutually responsive orientation between parents and their young children: Toward methodological advances in the science of relationships. *Developmental Psychology, 42*, 833–848.

Allen, J. P., Grande, L., Tan, J., & Loeb, E. (2018). Parent and peer predictors of change in attachment security from adolescence to adulthood. *Child Development, 89*, 1120–1132.

Almas, A. N., Grusec, J. E., & Tackett, J. L. (2011). Children's disclosure and secrecy: Links to maternal parenting characteristics and children's coping skills. *Social Development, 20*, 624–643.

Anderson, C. A., Shibuya, A., Ihori, N., Swing, E. L., Bushman, B. J., Sakamoto, A., . . . Saleem, M. (2010). Violent video game effects on aggression, empathy, and prosocial behavior in Eastern and Western countries: A meta-analytic review. *Psychological Bulletin, 136*, 151–173.

Arsenio, W. F. (1988). Children's conceptions of the situational affective consequences of sociomoral events. *Child Development, 59*, 1611–1622.

Arsenio, W. (2014). Moral emotion attributions and aggression. In M. Killen & J. Smetana (Eds.), *Handbook of moral development* (2nd ed., pp. 235–255). New York: Psychology Press.

Assor, A., Roth, G., & Deci, E. L. (2004). The emotional costs of parents' conditional regard: A self-determination theory analysis. *Journal of Personality, 72*, 47–88.

Atkin, A. L., Yoo, H. C., & Yeh, C. J. (2018). What types of racial messages protect Asian American adolescents from discrimination?: A latent interaction model. *Journal of Counseling Psychology.* [Epub ahead of print]

Avinun, R., & Knafo-Noam, A. (2015). Socialization, genetics, and their interplay in development. In J. E. Grusec & P. D. Hastings (Eds.), *Handbook of socialization: Theory and research* (2nd ed., pp. 347–371). New York: Guilford Press.

Awong, T., Grusec, J. E., & Sorenson, A. (2008). Respect-based control and anger as determinants of children's socio-emotional development. *Social Development, 17*, 941–959.

Baer, J. C., & Martinez, C. D. (2006). Child maltreatment and insecure attachment: A meta-analysis. *Journal of Reproductive and Infant Psychology, 24*, 187–197.

Baird, A. A. (2008). Adolescent moral reasoning: The integration of emotion and cognition. *Moral Psychology, 3*, 323–342.

Baldwin, A. L. (1955). *Behavior and development in childhood.* New York: Dryden Press.

Baldwin, J. M. (1906). *Thought and things: A study of the development and meaning of thought, or genetic logic.* London: Swan Sonnenschein.

Bandura, A. (1977). *Social learning theory.* Englewood Cliffs, NJ: Prentice-Hall.

Bandura, A. (1986). *Social foundations of thought and action: A social cognitive theory.* Englewood Cliffs, NJ: Prentice-Hall.

Bandura, A. (1999). Moral disengagement in the perpetration of inhumanities. *Personality and Social Psychology Review, 3*, 193–209.

Bandura, A., Grusec, J. E., & Menlove, F. L. (1967). Vicarious extinction of avoidance behavior. *Journal of Personality and Social Psychology, 5*, 16–23.

Bandura, A., & McDonald, F. J. (1963). Influence of social reinforcement and the behavior of models in shaping children's moral judgment. *Journal of Abnormal and Social Psychology, 67*, 274–281.

Bandura, A., Ross, D., & Ross, S. A. (1961). Transmission of aggression through imitation of aggressive models. *Journal of Abnormal and Social Psychology, 63*, 575–582.

Bandura, A., Ross, D., & Ross, S. A. (1963). Imitation of film-mediated aggressive models. *Journal of Abnormal and Social Psychology, 66*, 3–11.

Bandura, A., & Walters, R. H. (1963). *Social learning and personality development.* New York: Holt, Rinehart & Winston.

Barber, B. K. (1996). Parental psychological control: Revisiting a neglected construct. *Child Development, 67*, 3296–3319.

Barber, B. K., & Harmon, E. L. (2002). Violating the self: Parental psychological control of children and adolescents. In B. K. Barber (Ed.), *Intrusive parenting: How psychological control affects children and adolescents* (pp. 15–52). Washington, DC: American Psychological Association.

Barden, R. C., Zelko, F. A., Duncan, S. W., & Masters, J. C. (1980). Children's consensual knowledge about the experiential determinants of emotion. *Journal of Personality and Social Psychology, 39,* 968–976.

Barni, D., Ranieri, S., Scabini, E., & Rosnati, R. (2011). Value transmission in the family: Do adolescents accept the values their parents want to transmit? *Journal of Moral Education, 40,* 105–121.

Bates, J. E., & Pettit, G. S. (2015). Temperament, parenting, and social development. In J. E. Grusec & P. D. Hastings (Eds.), *Handbook of socialization: Theory and research* (2nd ed., pp. 372–397). New York: Guilford Press.

Batson, C. D., Futz, J., & Schoenrade, P. A. (1987). Distress and empathy: Two qualitatively distinct vicarious emotions with different motivational consequences. *Journal of Personality, 55,* 19–39.

Baumrind, D. (1971). Current patterns of parental authority. *Developmental Psychology Monographs, 4,* 1–103.

Baumrind, D. (2012). Differentiating between confrontive and coercive kinds of parental power-assertive disciplinary practices. *Human Development, 55,* 35–51.

Baumrind, D., Larzelere, R., & Cowan, P. (2002). Ordinary physical punishment: Is it harmful? Comment on Gershoff (2002). *Psychological Bulletin, 128,* 580–589.

Baumrind, D., & Thompson, R. A. (2002). The ethics of parenting. In M. H. Bornstein (Ed.), *Handbook of parenting: Practical issues in parenting* (pp. 3–34). Mahwah, NJ: Erlbaum.

Behne, T., Carpenter, M., & Tomasello, M. (2005). One-year-olds comprehend the communicative intentions behind gestures in a hiding game. *Developmental Science, 8,* 492–499.

Bell, R. Q., & Harper, I. V. (1977). *Child effects on adults.* Hillsdale, NJ: Erlbaum.

Belsky, J. (1999). Interactional and contextual determinants of attachment security. In J. Cassidy & P. R. Shaver (Eds.), *Handbook of attachment: Theory, research, and clinical applications* (pp. 249–264). New York: Guilford Press.

Belsky, J., & Cassidy, J. (1994). Attachment: Theory and evidence. In M. Rutte & D. Hay (Eds.), *Development through life: A handbook for clinicians* (pp. 373–402). Oxford, UK: Blackwell.

Benish-Weisman, M. (2015). The interplay between values and aggression in adolescence: A longitudinal study. *Developmental Psychology, 51,* 677–687.

Bennett, M., & Sani, F. (2008). Children's subjective identification with social groups: A group-reference effect approach. *British Journal of Developmental Psychology, 26,* 381–387.

Bergmeier, H., Aksan, N., McPhie, S., Fuller-Tyszkiewicz, M., Baur, L., Milgrom, J., . . . Skouteris, H. (2016). Mutually Responsive Orientation: A novel observational assessment of mother–child mealtime interactions. *Appetite, 105,* 400–409.

Berkowitz, M. W., Gibbs, J. C., & Broughton, J. M. (1980). The relation of moral judgment stage disparity to developmental effects of peer dialogues. *Merrill–Palmer Quarterly, 26,* 341–357.

Bernier, A., Carlson, S. M., & Whipple, N. (2010). From external regulation to self-regulation: Early parenting precursors of young children's executive functioning. *Child Development, 81*, 326–339.

Blasi, A. (2004). Moral functioning: Moral understanding and personality. In D. K. Lapsley & D. Narvaez (Eds.), *Moral development, self, and identity* (pp. 335–347). Mahwah, NJ: Erlbaum.

Blatz, W. E. (1944). *Understanding the young child.* New York: Morrow.

Boehm, C. (2000). Conflict and the evolution of social control. *Journal of Consciousness Studies, 7*, 79–101.

Bornstein, M. (2007). On the significance of social relationships in the development of children's earliest symbolic play: An ecological perspective. In A. Göncü & S. Gaskins (Eds.), *Play and development: Evolutionary, sociocultural, and functional perspectives* (pp. 101–130). Mahwah, NJ: Erlbaum.

Bornstein, M. H., & Tamis-Lemonda, C. S. (1997). Maternal responsiveness and infant mental abilities: Specific predictive relations. *Infant Behavior and Development, 20*, 283–296.

Bowlby, J. (1944). Forty-four juvenile thieves: Their characters and home lives. *International Journal of Psychoanalysis, 25*, 19–52.

Bowlby, J. (1969). *Attachment and loss: Vol. 1. Attachment.* New York: Basic Books.

Bowlby, J. (1973). *Attachment and loss: Vol. 2. Separation: Anxiety and anger.* New York: Basic Books.

Bowlby, J. (1979). *The making and breaking of affectional bonds.* London: Tavistock.

Bowlby, J. (1982). *Attachment and loss: Vol. 1. Attachment* (2nd ed.). New York: Basic Books.

Bowlby, J., & Robertson, J. (1953). A two-year-old goes to hospital. *Proceedings of the Royal Society of Medicine, 46*, 425–427.

Brehm, S. S., & Brehm, J. W. (1981). *Psychological reactance: A theory of freedom and control.* New York: Academic Press.

Bretherton, I. (1992). The origins of attachment theory: John Bowlby and Mary Ainsworth. *Developmental Psychology, 28*, 759–775.

Bretherton, I., Ridgeway, D., & Cassidy, J. (1990). Assessing internal working models of the attachment relationship. In M. T. Greenberg, D. Cicchetti, & E. M. Cummings (Eds.), *Attachment in the preschool years: Theory, research, and intervention* (pp. 273–308). Chicago: University of Chicago Press.

Brewer, M. B. (1999). The psychology of prejudice: Ingroup love and outgroup hate? *Journal of Social Issues, 55*, 429–444.

Brody, G. H., & Flor, D. L. (1998). Maternal resources, parenting practices, and child competence in rural, single-parent African American families. *Child Development, 69*, 803–816.

Brownell, C. A., & Early Social Development Research Lab. (2016). Prosocial behavior in infancy: The role of socialization. *Child Development Perspectives, 10*, 222–227.

Brownell, C. A., Svetlova, M., Anderson, R., Nichols, S. R., & Drummond, J. (2013). Socialization of early prosocial behavior: Parents' talk about emotions is associated with sharing and helping in toddlers. *Infancy, 18*, 91–119.

Buchner, A., Bell, R., Mehl, B., & Musch, J. (2009). No enhanced recognition memory, but better source memory for faces of cheaters. *Evolution and Human Behavior, 30*, 212–224.

Bugental, D. B. (2000). Acquisition of algorithms of social life: A domain-based approach. *Psychological Bulletin, 26*, 187–209.

Bugental, D. B., & Goodnow, J. J. (1998). Socialization processes. In W. Damon (Series Ed.) & N. Eisenberg (Vol. Ed.), *Handbook of child psychology: Vol. 3. Social, emotional, and personality development* (5th ed., pp. 389–462). New York: Wiley.

Bugental, D. B., & Grusec, J. E. (2006). Socialization processes. In W. Damon & R. M. Lerner (Series Eds.) & N. Eisenberg (Vol. Ed.), *Handbook of child psychology: Vol. 3. Social, emotional, and personality development* (6th ed., pp. 366–428). Hoboken, NJ: Wiley.

Bugental, D. E., Kaswan, J. W., Love, L. R., & Fox, M. N. (1970). Child versus adult perception of evaluative messages in verbal, vocal, and visual channels. *Developmental Psychology, 2*, 367–375.

Bushman, B. J., & Huesmann, L. R. (2010). Aggression. In S. T. Fiske, D. T. Gilbert, & G. Lindzey (Eds.), *Handbook of social psychology* (5th ed., Vol. 2, pp. 833–863). Hoboken, NJ: Wiley.

Cairns, R. B. (1979). *Social development: The origins and plasticity of interchanges.* San Francisco: Freeman.

Carlo, G., Roesch, S. C., Knight, G. P., & Koller, S. H. (2001). Between- or within-culture variation?: Culture group as a moderator of the relations between individual differences and resource allocation preferences. *Journal of Applied Developmental Psychology, 22*, 559–579.

Cassidy, J., & Shaver, P. R. (Eds.). (2016). *Handbook of attachment: Theory, research, and clinical applications* (3rd ed.). New York: Guilford Press.

Chao, R. K. (1994). Beyond parental control and authoritarian parenting style: Understanding Chinese parenting through the cultural notion of training. *Child Development, 65*, 1111–1119.

Chao, R. K. (2001). Extending research on the consequences of parenting style for Chinese Americans and European Americans. *Child Development, 72*, 1832–1843.

Chaparro, M. P., & Grusec, J. E. (2015). Parent and adolescent intentions to disclose and links to positive social behavior. *Journal of Family Psychology, 29*, 49–58.

Chaparro, M. P., & Grusec, J. E. (2016). Neuroticism moderates the relation between parenting and empathy and between empathy and prosocial behavior. *Merrill–Palmer Quarterly, 62*, 105–128.

Colby, A., Kohlberg, L., Gibbs, J., Lieberman, M., Fischer, K., & Saltzstein, H. D. (1983). A longitudinal study of moral judgment. *Monographs of the Society for Research in Child Development, 48*(1–2), 1–124.

Collier, K. M., Coyne, S. M., Rasmussen, E. E., Hawkins, A. J., Padilla-Walker, L. M., Erickson, S. E., & Memmott-Elison, M. K. (2016). Does parental mediation of media influence child outcomes?: A meta-analysis on media time, aggression, substance use, and sexual behavior. *Developmental Psychology, 52*, 798–812.

Cornell, A. H., & Frick, P. J. (2007). The moderating effects of parenting styles in the association between behavioral inhibition and parent-reported guilt and empathy in preschool children. *Journal of Clinical Child and Adolescent Psychology, 36*, 305–318.

Cosmides, L., & Tooby, J. (1992). Cognitive adaptations for social exchange. In J. H. Barkow, L. Cosmides, & J. Tooby (Eds.), *The adapted mind: Evolutionary psychology and the generation of culture* (pp. 163–228). New York: Oxford University Press.

Coyne, S. M., Padilla-Walker, L., Holmgren, H. G., Davis, E. J., Collier, K. M., Memmott-Elison, M., & Hawkins, A. J. (2018). A meta-analysis of prosocial media on prosocial behavior, aggression, and empathic concern: A multidimensional approach. *Developmental Psychology, 54*, 331–347.

Criss, M. M., Morris, A. S., Ponce-Garcia, E., Cui, L., & Silk, J. S. (2016). Pathways to adaptive emotion regulation among adolescents from low-income families. *Family Relations, 65*, 517–529.

Crouter, A. C., & Head, M. R. (2002). Parental monitoring and knowledge of children. In M. H. Bornstein (Ed.), *Handbook of parenting: Being and becoming a parent* (pp. 461–483). Mahwah, NJ: Erlbaum.

Crouter, A. C., Helms-Erikson, H., Updegraff, K., & McHale, S. M. (1999). Conditions underlying parents' knowledge about children's daily lives in middle childhood: Between- and within-family comparisons. *Child Development, 70*, 246–259.

Dadds, M. R., Sheffield, J. K., & Holbeck, J. F. (1990). An examination of the differential relationship of marital discord to parents' discipline strategies for boys and girls. *Journal of Abnormal Child Psychology, 18*, 121–129.

Dahl, A., & Campos, J. J. (2013). Domain differences in early social interactions. *Child Development, 84*, 817–825.

Dahl, A., Sherlock, B. R., Campos, J. J., & Theunissen, F. (2014). Mothers' tone of voice depends on the nature of infants' transgressions. *Emotion, 14*, 651–665.

Darling, N., Cumsille, P., Caldwell, L. L., & Dowdy, B. (2006). Predictors of adolescents' disclosure to parents and perceived parental knowledge: Between- and within-person differences. *Journal of Youth and Adolescence, 35*, 659–670.

Darling, N., & Steinberg, L. (1993). Parenting style as context: An integrative model. *Psychological Bulletin, 113*, 487–496.

Davidov, M. (2013). The socialization of self-regulation from a domains perspective. In G. Seebaß, M. Schmitz, & P. M. Gollwitzer (Eds.), *Acting intentionally and its limits: Individuals, groups, institutions* (pp. 223–244). Berlin, Germany: DeGruyter.

Davidov, M., & Grusec, J. E. (2006a). Untangling the links of parental responsiveness to distress and warmth to child outcomes. *Child Development, 77*, 44–58.

Davidov, M., & Grusec, J. E. (2006b). Multiple pathways to compliance: Mothers' willingness to cooperate and knowledge of their children's reactions to discipline. *Journal of Family Psychology, 20,* 705–708.

Davidov, M., Grusec, J. E., & Wolfe, J. L. (2012). Mothers' knowledge of their children's evaluations of discipline: The role of type of discipline and misdeed, and parenting practices. *Merrill–Palmer Quarterly, 58,* 314–340.

Davidov, M., Tuvia, S. M., Polacheck, N., & Grusec, J. E. (2018). *Two forms of mother–child reciprocity and their links to children's cooperativeness.* Unpublished manuscript, Hebrew University, New York.

Deater-Deckard, K., Atzaba-Poria, N., & Pike, A. (2004). Mother– and father–child mutuality in Anglo and Indian British families: A link with lower externalizing problems. *Journal of Abnormal Child Psychology, 32,* 609–620.

Deater-Deckard, K., Dodge, K. A., Bates, J. E., & Pettit, G. S. (1996). Physical discipline among African American and European American mothers: Links to children's externalizing behaviors. *Developmental Psychology, 32,* 1065–1072.

Deater-Deckard, K., Ivy, L., & Petrill, S. A. (2006). Maternal warmth moderates the link between physical punishment and child externalizing problems: A parent–offspring behavior genetic analysis. *Parenting: Science and Practice, 6,* 59–78.

Deater-Deckard, K., & O'Connor, T. G. (2000). Parent–child mutuality in early childhood: Two behavioral genetic studies. *Developmental Psychology, 36,* 561–570.

Deater-Deckard, K., & Petrill, S. A. (2004). Parent–child dyadic mutuality and child behavior problems: An investigation of gene–environment processes. *Journal of Child Psychology and Psychiatry, 45,* 1171–1179.

Decety, J. (2011). Dissecting the neural mechanisms mediating empathy. *Emotion Review, 3,* 92–108.

Decety, J., Michalska, K. J., & Kinzler, K. D. (2011). The developmental neuroscience of moral sensitivity. *Emotion Review, 3,* 305–307.

Deci, E. L., Koestner, R., & Ryan, R. M. (1999). A meta-analytic review of experiments examining the effects of extrinsic rewards on intrinsic motivation. *Psychological Bulletin, 125,* 627–668.

Deci, E. L., & Ryan, R. M. (1985). *Intrinsic motivation and self-motivation in human behavior.* New York: Plenum Press.

Degnan, K. A., Henderson, H. A., Fox, N. A., & Rubin, K. H. (2008). Predicting social wariness in middle childhood: The moderating roles of childcare history, maternal personality and maternal behavior. *Social Development, 17,* 471–487.

Dijkstra, J. K., & Veenstra, R. (2011). Peer relations. In B. B. Brown & M. J. Prinstein (Eds.), *Encyclopedia of adolescence* (Vol. 2, pp. 255–259). San Diego, CA: Academic Press.

Dishion, T. J., Patterson, G. R., & Kavanagh, K. A. (1992). An experimental test of the coercion model: Linking theory, measurement, and intervention. In J. McCord & R. E. Tremblay (Eds.), *Preventing antisocial behavior: Interventions from birth through adolescence* (pp. 253–282). New York: Guilford Press.

Dishion, T. J., Véronneau, M. H., & Myers, M. W. (2010). Cascading peer dynamics underlying the progression from problem behavior to violence in early to late adolescence *Development and Psychopathology, 22*, 603–619.

Dollard, J., Doob, L., Miller, N. E., Mowrer, O. H., & Sears, R. R. (1939). *Frustration and aggression*. New Haven, CT: Yale University Press.

Dozier, M., Stovall, K. C., Albus, K. E., & Bates, B. (2001). Attachment for infants in foster care: The role of caregiver state of mind. *Child Development, 72*, 1467–1477.

Dunfield, K. A., & Kuhlmeier, V. A. (2010). Intention-mediated selective helping in infancy. *Psychological Science, 21*, 523–527.

Dunham, Y., Baron, A. S., & Banaji, M. R. (2008). The development of implicit intergroup cognition. *Trends in Cognitive Sciences, 12*, 248–253.

Dunn, J., & Hughes, C. (2014). Family talk about moral issues: The toddler and preschool years. In C. Wainryb & H. Recchia (Eds.), *Talking about right and wrong: Parent–child conversations as contexts for moral development* (pp. 21–43). Cambridge, UK: Cambridge University Press.

Dweck, C. S. (1975). The role of expectations and attributions in the alleviation of learned helplessness. *Journal of Personality and Social Psychology, 31*, 674–685.

Dweck, C. S., & Reppucci, N. D. (1973). Learned helplessness and reinforcement responsibility in children. *Journal of Personality and Social Psychology, 25*, 109–116.

Egeland, B., Jacobvitz, D., & Sroufe, L. A. (1988). Breaking the cycle of abuse. *Child Development, 59*, 1080–1088.

Eisenberg, N. (2000). Emotion, regulation, and moral development. *Annual Review of Psychology, 51*, 665–697.

Eisenberg, N., Fabes, R. A., & Spinrad, T. L. (2006). Prosocial development. In W. Damon & R. M. Lerner (Series Eds.) & N. Eisenberg (Vol. Ed.), *Handbook of child psychology: Vol. 3. Social, emotional, and personality development* (6th ed., pp. 646–718). Hoboken, NJ: Wiley.

Eisenberg, N., Lennon, R., & Roth, K. (1983). Prosocial development: A longitudinal study. *Developmental Psychology, 19*, 846–855.

Eisenberg, N., Spinrad, T. L., & Knafo-Noam, A. (2015). Prosocial development. In R. M. Lerner (Series Ed.) & M. E. Lamb (Vol. Ed.). *Handbook of child psychology and developmental processes: Vol. 3. Socioemotional processes* (7th ed., pp. 610–658). Hoboken, NJ: Wiley.

Eisenberg, N., Spinrad, T. L., Taylor, Z. E., & Liew, J. (2017). Relations of inhibition and emotion-related parenting to young children's prosocial and vicariously induced distress behavior. *Child Development*. [Epub ahead of print]

Eisenberg-Berg, N., & Geisheker, E. (1979). Content of preachings and power of the model/preacher: The effect on children's generosity. *Developmental Psychology, 15*, 168–175.

Ellison, C. G., Musick, M. A., & Holden, G. W. (2011). Does conservative Protestantism moderate the association between corporal punishment and child outcomes? *Journal of Marriage and Family, 73*, 946–961.

Evans, M. B., Allan, V., Erickson, K., Martin, L. J., Budziszewski, R., & Côté,

J. (2016). Are all sport activities equal?: A systematic review of how youth psychosocial experiences vary across differing sport activities. *British Journal of Sports Medicine, 51*, 169–176.

Fearon, R. P., Bakermans-Kranenburg, M. J., van IJzendoorn, M. H., Lapsley, A. M., & Roisman, G. I. (2010). The significance of insecure attachment and disorganization in the development of children's externalizing behavior: A meta-analytic study. *Child Development, 81*, 435–456.

Feldman, R. (2012). Parent–infant synchrony: A biobehavioral model of mutual influences in the formation of affiliative bonds. *Monographs of the Society for Research in Child Development, 77*(2), 42–51.

Feldman, R., Granat, A., Pariente, C., Kanety, H., Kuint, J., & Gilboa-Schechtman, E. (2009). Maternal depression and anxiety across the postpartum year and infant social engagement, fear regulation, and stress reactivity. *Journal of the American Academy of Child and Adolescent Psychiatry, 48*, 919–927.

Ferguson, T. J., & Stegge, H. (1998). Measuring guilt in children: A rose by any other name still has thorns. In J. Bybee (Ed.), *Guilt and children* (pp. 19–74). San Diego, CA: Academic Press.

Fiese, B. H., Tomcho, T. J., Douglas, M., Josephs, K., Poltrock, S., & Baker, T. (2002). A review of 50 years of research on naturally occurring family routines and rituals: Cause for celebration? *Journal of Family Psychology, 16*, 381–390.

Fisher, J. D., Nadler, A., & Whitcher-Alagna, S. (1982). Recipient reactions to aid. *Psychological Bulletin, 91*, 27–54.

Fivush, R. (2001). Owning experience: The development of subjective perspective in autobiographical memory. In C. Moore & K. Lemmon (Eds.), *The self in time: Developmental perspectives* (pp. 35–52). Mahwah, NJ: Erlbaum.

Fivush, R. (2004). The silenced self: Constructing self from memories spoken and unspoken. In D. Beike, J. Lampinen, & D. Behrend (Eds.), *The self and memory* (pp. 75–94). New York: Psychology Press.

Fivush, R., Bohanek, J., Robertson, R., & Duke, M. (2004). Family narratives and the development of children's emotional well-being. In M. W. Pratt & B. H. Fiese (Eds.), *Family stories and the life course: Across time and generations* (pp. 55–76). Mahwah, NJ: Erlbaum.

Fivush, R., Bohanek, J. G., & Zaman, W. (2011). Personal and intergenerational narratives in relation to adolescents' well-being. In T. Habermas (Ed.), *The development of autobiographical reasoning in adolescence and beyond* (pp. 45–57). San Francisco: Jossey-Bass.

Fivush, R., Haden, C. A., & Reese, E. (2006). Elaborating on elaborations: Role of maternal reminiscing style in cognitive and socioemotional development. *Child Development, 77*, 1568–1588.

Fivush, R., Merrill, N., & Marin, K. (2014). Voice and power: Constructing moral agency through personal and intergenerational narratives. In C. Weinryb & H. Recchia (Eds.), *Talking about right and wrong: Parent–child conversations as contexts for moral development* (pp. 270–297). Cambridge, UK: Cambridge University Press.

Fivush, R., & Wang, Q. (2005). Emotion talk in mother–child conversations of the shared past: The effects of culture, gender, and event valence. *Journal of Cognition and Development, 6*, 489–506.

Fletcher, A. C., Steinberg, L., & Williams-Wheeler, M. (2004). Parental influences on adolescent problem behavior: Revisiting Stattin and Kerr. *Child Development, 75*, 781–796.

Fonagy, P., Steele, H., & Steele, M. (1991). Maternal representations of attachment during pregnancy predict the organization of infant–mother attachment at one year of age. *Child Development, 62*, 891–905.

Fox, N. A., & Davidson, R. J. (1987). Electroencephalogram asymmetry in response to the approach of a stranger and maternal separation in 10-month-old infants. *Developmental Psychology, 23*, 233–240.

Fraser, A. M., Padilla-Walker, L. M., Coyne, S. M., Nelson, L. J., & Stockdale, L. A. (2012). Associations between violent video gaming, empathic concern, and prosocial behavior toward strangers, friends, and family members. *Journal of Youth and Adolescence, 41*, 636–649.

Freedman, J. L. (1965). Long-term behavioral effects of cognitive dissonance. *Journal of Experimental Social Psychology, 1*, 145–155.

Freud, S. (1930). *Das Unbehagen in der Kultur [Civilization and its discontents]*. Vienna: Psychoanalytischer Verlag Wien.

Frodi, A., & Thompson, R. (1985). Infants' affective responses in the Strange Situation: Effects of prematurity and of quality of attachment. *Child Development, 56*, 1280–1290.

Garner, P. W., Dunsmore, J. C., & Southam-Gerrow, M. (2008). Mother–child conversations about emotions: Linkages to child aggression and prosocial behavior. *Social Development, 17*, 259–277.

Gath, M., & Grusec, J. E. (2018). *Mothers' moral identity and their warmth and involvement: Relation to adolescent prosociality*. Unpublished manuscript, University of Toronto, Toronto, ON, Canada.

Gauvain, M., & Perez, S. M. (2015). The socialization of cognition. In J. E. Grusec & P. D. Hastings (Eds.), *Handbook of socialization: Theory and research* (2nd ed., pp. 566–589). New York: Guilford Press.

Ge, X., Conger, R. D., Cadoret, R. J., Neiderhiser, J. M., Yates, W., Troughton, E., & Stewart, M. A. (1996). The developmental interface between nature and nurture: A mutual influence model of child antisocial behavior and parent behaviors. *Developmental Psychology, 32*, 574–589.

George, C., Kaplan, N., & Main, M. (1985). *The Adult Attachment Interview*. Unpublished manuscript, University of California, Berkeley, CA.

George, C., & Solomon, J. (1996). Representational models of relationships: Links between caregiving and attachment. *Infant Mental Health Journal, 17*, 198–216.

Gershoff, E. T. (2002). Corporal punishment by parents and associated child behaviors and experiences: A meta-analytic and theoretical review. *Psychological Bulletin, 128*, 539–579.

Gershoff, E. T., & Grogan-Kaylor, A. (2016). Spanking and child outcomes:

Old controversies and new meta-analyses. *Journal of Family Psychology, 30,* 453–469.

Gershoff, E. T., Grogan-Kaylor, A., Lansford, J. E., Chang, L., Zelli, A., Deater-Deckard, K., & Dodge, K. A. (2010). Parent discipline practices in an international sample: Associations with child behaviors and moderation by perceived normativeness. *Child Development, 81,* 487–502.

Gewirtz, J. L., & Boyd, E. F. (1977). Does maternal responding imply reduced infant crying?: A critique of the 1972 Bell and Ainsworth report. *Child Development, 48,* 1200–1207.

Gianino, A., & Tronick, E. Z. (1988). The mutual regulation model: The infant's self and interactive regulation and coping and defensive capacities. In T. M. Field, P. M. McCabe, & N. Schneiderman (Eds.), *Stress and coping across development* (pp. 47–68). Hillsdale, NJ: Erlbaum.

Gibbs, J. C., Basinger, K. S., Grime, R. L., & Snarey, J. R. (2007). Moral judgment development across cultures: Revisiting Kohlberg's universality claims. *Developmental Review, 27*(4), 443–500.

Goldberg, S., Grusec, J. E., & Jenkins, J. M. (1999). Confidence in protection: Arguments for a narrow definition of attachment. *Journal of Family Psychology, 13,* 475–483.

Goodnow, J. J. (1988). Children's household work: Its nature and functions. *Psychological Bulletin, 103,* 5–26.

Goodnow, J. J. (1997). Parenting and the transmission and internalization of values: From social-cultural perspectives to within-family analyses. In J. E. Grusec & L. Kuczynski (Eds.), *Parenting and children's internalization of values: A handbook of contemporary theory* (pp. 333–361). New York: Wiley.

Goossens, F. A., & van IJzendoorn, M. H. (1990). Quality of infants' attachments to professional caregivers: Relation to infant–parent attachment and daycare characteristics. *Child Development, 61,* 832–837.

Gottman, J. M., Katz, L. F., & Hooven, C. (1996). Parental meta-emotion philosophy and the emotional life of families: Theoretical models and preliminary data. *Journal of Family Psychology, 10,* 243–268.

Grazzani, I., Ornaghi, V., Agliati, A., & Brazzelli, E. (2016). How to foster toddlers' mental-state talk, emotion understanding, and prosocial behavior: A conversation-based intervention at nursery school. *Infancy, 21,* 199–227.

Greitemeyer, T., Hollingdale, J., & Traut-Mattausch, E. (2015). Changing the track in music and misogyny: Listening to music with pro-equality lyrics improves attitudes and behavior toward women. *Psychology of Popular Media Culture, 4,* 56–67.

Groh, A. M., Fearon, R. P., Bakermans-Kranenburg, M. J., van IJzendoorn, M. H., Steele, R. D., & Roisman, G. I. (2014). The significance of attachment security for children's social competence with peers: A meta-analytic study. *Attachment and Human Development, 16,* 103–136.

Groh, A. M., Narayan, A. J., Bakermans-Kranenburg, M. J., Roisman, G. I., Vaughn, B. E., Fearon, R. M. P., & van IJzendoorn, M. H. (2017).

Attachment and temperament in the early life course: A meta-analytic review. *Child Development, 88,* 770–795.

Grolnick, W. S., Deci, E. L., & Ryan, R. M. (1997). Internalization within the family: The self-determination theory perspective. In J. E. Grusec & L. Kuczynski (Eds.), *Parenting and children's internalization of values: A handbook of contemporary theory* (pp. 135–161). New York: Wiley.

Grossmann, K., Grossmann, K. E., Spangler, G., Suess, G., & Unzner, L. (1985). Maternal sensitivity and newborns' orientation responses as related to quality of attachment in northern Germany. *Monographs of the Society for Research in Child Development, 50*(1–2), 233–256.

Grusec, J. E. (1991). Socializing concern for others in the home. *Developmental Psychology, 27,* 338–342.

Grusec, J. E. (1992). Social learning theory and developmental psychology: The legacy of Robert Sears and Albert Bandura. *Developmental Psychology, 28,* 776–786.

Grusec, J. E., & Davidov, M. (2007). Socialization in the family: The roles of parents. In J. E. Grusec & P. D. Hastings (Eds.), *Handbook of socialization: Theory and research* (pp. 284–308). New York: Guilford Press.

Grusec, J. E., & Davidov, M. (2010). Integrating different perspectives on socialization theory and research: A domain-specific approach. *Child Development, 81,* 687–709.

Grusec, J. E., Dix, T., & Mills, R. (1982). The effects of type, severity, and victim of children's transgressions on maternal discipline. *Canadian Journal of Behavioural Science, 14,* 276–289.

Grusec, J. E., & Goodnow, J. J. (1994). Impact of parental discipline methods on the child's internalization of values: A reconceptualization of current points of view. *Developmental Psychology, 30,* 4–19.

Grusec, J. E., Goodnow, J. J., & Cohen, L. (1997) Household work and the development of children's concern for others. *Developmental Psychology, 32,* 999–1007.

Grusec, J. E., Goodnow, J. J., & Kuczynski, L. (2000). New directions in analyses of parenting contributions to children's acquisition of values. *Child Development, 71,* 205–211.

Grusec, J. E., & Kuczynski, L. (1980). Direction of effect in socialization: A comparison of the parent's versus the child's behavior as determinants of disciplinary techniques. *Developmental Psychology, 16,* 1–9.

Grusec, J. E., & Redler, E. (1980). Attribution, reinforcement, and altruism: A developmental analysis. *Developmental Psychology, 16,* 525–534.

Gunnar, M. R. (2000). Early adversity and the development of stress reactivity and regulation. In C. A. Nelson (Ed.), *Minnesota Symposia on Child Psychology: Vol. 31. The effects of early adversity on neurobehavioral development* (pp. 163–200). Mahwah, NJ: Erlbaum.

Gunnar, M. R., Morison, S. J., Chisholm, K. I. M., & Schuder, M. (2001). Salivary cortisol levels in children adopted from Romanian orphanages. *Development and Psychopathology, 13,* 611–628.

Gunnoe, M. L., Hetherington, E. M., & Reiss, D. (2006). Differential impact of fathers' authoritarian parenting on early adolescent adjustment in conservative Protestant versus other families. *Journal of Family Psychology, 20,* 589–596.

Halgunseth, L. C., Perkins, D. F., Lippold, M. A., & Nix, R. L. (2013). Delinquent-oriented attitudes mediate the relation between parental inconsistent discipline and early adolescent behavior. *Journal of Family Psychology, 27,* 293–302.

Hamlin, J. K. (2014). The origins of human morality: Complex socio-moral evaluations by preverbal infants. In J. Decety & Y. Christen (Eds.), *New frontiers in social neuroscience* (pp. 165–188). Cham, Switzerland: Springer.

Hamlin, J. K., & Wynn, K. (2011). Young infants prefer prosocial to antisocial others. *Cognitive Development, 26,* 30–39.

Hammond, S. I., & Carpendale, J. I. (2015). Helping children help: The relation between maternal scaffolding and children's early help. *Social Development, 24,* 367–383.

Harkness, S., & Super, C. M. (Eds.). (1996). *Parents' cultural belief systems: Their origins, expressions, and consequences.* New York: Guilford Press.

Harlow, H. F. (1958). The nature of love. *American Psychologist, 13,* 673–685.

Harlow, H. F., & Zimmermann, R. R. (1958). The development of affective responsiveness in infant monkeys. *Proceedings of the American Philosophical Society, 102,* 501–509.

Harrist, A. W., Pettit, G. S., Dodge, K. A., & Bates, J. E. (1994). Dyadic synchrony in mother–child interaction: Relation with children's subsequent kindergarten adjustment. *Family Relations, 43,* 417–424.

Harrist, A. W., & Waugh, R. M. (2002). Dyadic synchrony: Its structure and function in children's development. *Developmental Review, 22,* 555–592.

Hastings, P., & Grusec, J. E. (1997). Conflict outcome as a function of parental accuracy in perceiving child cognitions and affect. *Social Development, 6,* 76–90.

Hastings, P. D., Kahle, S., & Nuselovici, J. M. (2014). How well socially wary preschoolers fare over time depends on their parasympathetic regulation and socialization. *Child Development, 85,* 1586–1600.

Hastings, P. D., Miller, J. G., & Troxel, N. R. (2015). Making good: The socialization of children's prosocial development. In J. E. Grusec & P. D. Hastings (Eds.), *Handbook of socialization: Theory and research* (2nd ed., pp. 637–660). New York: Guilford Press.

Helwig, C. C. (2006). The development of personal autonomy throughout cultures. *Cognitive Development, 21,* 458–473.

Helwig, C. C., To, S., Wang, Q., Liu, C., & Yang, S. (2014). Judgments and reasoning about parental discipline involving induction and psychological control in China and Canada. *Child Development, 85,* 1150–1167.

Henderson, D. L., & May, J. P. (2005). *Exploring culturally diverse literature for children and adolescents: Learning to listen in new ways.* Boston: Pearson Allyn & Bacon.

Hess, R. D., Kashiwagi, K., Azuma, H., Price, G. G., & Dickson, W. P. (1980). Maternal expectations for mastery of developmental tasks in Japan and the United States. *International Journal of Psychology, 15,* 259–271.

Hoeve, M., Dubas, J. S., Eichelsheim, V. I., van der Laan, P. H., Smeenk, W., & Gerris, J. R. (2009). The relationship between parenting and delinquency: A meta-analysis. *Journal of Abnormal Child Psychology, 37,* 749–775.

Hoffman, M. L. (1970a). Conscience, personality, and socialization techniques. *Human Development, 13*(2), 90–126.

Hoffman, M. L. (1970b). Moral development. In P. H. Mussen (Ed.), *Carmichael's manual of child psychology* (Vol. 2, pp. 261–360). New York: Wiley.

Hoffman, M. L. (1982). Affect and moral development. *New Directions for Child and Adolescent Development, 1982*(16), 83–103.

Holden, G. W. (2002). Perspectives on the effects of corporal punishment: Comment on Gershoff (2002). *Psychological Bulletin, 128,* 590–595.

Huesmann, L. R., Moise-Titus, J., Podolski, C. L., & Eron, L. D. (2003). Longitudinal relations between children's exposure to TV violence and their aggressive and violent behavior in young adulthood: 1977–1992. *Developmental Psychology, 39,* 201–221.

Hughes, D., & Chen, L. (1997). When and what parents tell children about race: An examination of race-related socialization among African American families. *Applied Developmental Science, 1,* 200–214.

Im-Bolter, N., Anam, M., & Cohen, N. J. (2015). Mother–child synchrony and child problem behavior. *Journal of Child and Family Studies, 24,* 1876–1885.

Isabella, R. A., & Belsky, J. (1991). Interactional synchrony and the origins of infant–mother attachment: A replication study. *Child Development, 62,* 373–384.

Jaffee, S. R., Caspi, A., Moffitt, T. E., Polo-Tomas, M., Price, T. S., & Taylor, A. (2004). The limits of child effects: Evidence for genetically mediated child effects on corporal punishment but not on physical maltreatment. *Developmental Psychology, 40,* 1047–1058.

James, P. D. (1992). *The children of men.* New York: Knopf.

Joussemet, M., Landry, R., & Koestner, R. (2008). A self-determination theory perspective on parenting. *Canadian Psychology, 49,* 194–200.

Kagan, J. (1982). The emergence of self. *Journal of Child Psychology and Psychiatry, 23,* 363–381.

Kaplan, N., & Main, M. (1986). *Instructions for the classification of children's family drawings in terms of representation of attachment.* Unpublished manuscript, University of California, Berkeley, CA.

Kasser, T., & Ryan, R. M. (1996). Further examining the American dream: Differential correlates of intrinsic and extrinsic goals. *Personality and Social Psychology Bulletin, 22,* 280–287.

Keller, H., Lamm, B., Abels, M., Yovsi, R., Borke, J., Jensen, H., . . . Su, Y. (2006). Cultural models, socialization goals, and parenting ethnotheories: A multicultural analysis. *Journal of Cross-Cultural Psychology, 37,* 155–172.

Kerr, M., & Stattin, H. (2000). What parents know, how they know it, and several forms of adolescent adjustment: Further support for a reinterpretation of monitoring. *Developmental Psychology, 36,* 366–380.

Kerr, M., Stattin, H., & Burk, W. J. (2010). A reinterpretation of parental monitoring in longitudinal perspective. *Journal of Research on Adolescence, 20,* 39–64.

Kerr, M., Stattin, H., & Özdemir, M. (2012). Perceived parenting style and adolescent adjustment: Revisiting directions of effects and the role of parental knowledge. *Developmental Psychology, 48,* 1540–1553.

Kiel, E. J., & Buss, K. A. (2011). Prospective relations among fearful temperament, protective parenting, and social withdrawal: The role of maternal accuracy in a moderated mediation framework. *Journal of Abnormal Child Psychology, 39,* 953–966.

Kil, H., Grusec, J. E., & Chaparro, M. P. (2018). Maternal disclosure and adolescent prosocial behavior: The mediating roles of adolescent disclosure and coping. *Social Development, 27,* 652–664.

Kilgore, K., Snyder, J., & Lentz, C. (2000). The contribution of parental discipline, parental monitoring, and school risk to early-onset conduct problems in African American boys and girls. *Developmental Psychology, 36,* 835–845.

Killen, M., Breton, S., Ferguson, H., & Handler, K. (1994). Preschoolers' evaluations of teacher methods of intervention in social transgressions. *Merrill–Palmer Quarterly, 40,* 399–415.

Klein, M. (1952). The origins of transference. *International Journal of Psycho-Analysis, 33,* 433–438.

Klopfer, B., Ainsworth, M. D., Klopfer, W. G., & Holt, R. R. (1954). *Developments in the Rorschach technique: Vol. 1. Technique and theory.* Oxford, UK: World.

Klopfer, B., Ainsworth, M. D., Klopfer, W. G., & Holt, R. R. (1956). *Developments in the Rorschach technique: Vol. 2. Fields of application.* Oxford, UK: World.

Knafo, A., & Jaffee, S. R. (2013). Gene–environment correlation in developmental psychopathology. *Development and Psychopathology, 25,* 1–6.

Knafo, A., & Schwartz, S. H. (2003). Parenting and adolescents' accuracy in perceiving parental values. *Child Development, 74,* 595–611.

Kochanska, G. (1995). Children's temperament, mothers' discipline, and security of attachment: Multiple pathways to emerging internalization. *Child Development, 66,* 597–615.

Kochanska, G. (1997). Mutually responsive orientation between mothers and their young children: Implications for early socialization. *Child Development, 68,* 94–112.

Kochanska, G., Aksan, N., & Joy, M. E. (2007). Children's fearfulness as a moderator of parenting in early socialization: Two longitudinal studies. *Developmental Psychology, 43,* 222–237.

Kochanska, G., Aksan, N., Prisco, T. R., & Adams, E. E. (2008). Mother–child and father–child mutually responsive orientation in the first 2 years and children's outcomes at preschool age: Mechanisms of influence. *Child Development, 79,* 30–44.

Kochanska, G., & Kim, S. (2012). Toward a new understanding of legacy of early attachments for future antisocial trajectories: Evidence from two longitudinal studies. *Development and Psychopathology, 24,* 783–806.

Kochanska, G., Kim, S., Boldt, L. J., & Nordling, J. K. (2013). Promoting toddlers' positive social-emotional outcomes in low-income families: A play-based experimental study. *Journal of Clinical Child and Adolescent Psychology, 42,* 700–712.

Kohlberg, L. (1976). Moral stages and moralization: The cognitive-developmental approach. In T. Lickona (Ed.), *Moral development and behavior: Theory, research and social issues* (pp. 31–53). New York: Holt, Rinehart & Winston.

Koss, K. J., & Gunnar, M. R. (2018). Annual research review: Early adversity, the hypothalamic–pituitary–adrenocortical axis, and child psychopathology. *Journal of Child Psychology and Psychiatry, 59,* 327–346.

Krahé, B., & Möller, I. (2010). Longitudinal effects of media violence on aggression and empathy among German adolescents. *Journal of Applied Developmental Psychology, 31,* 401–409.

Kremer, K. P., Maynard, B. R., Polanin, J. R., Vaughn, M. G., & Sarteschi, C. M. (2015). Effects of after-school programs with at-risk youth on attendance and externalizing behaviors: A systematic review and meta-analysis. *Journal of Youth and Adolescence, 44,* 616–636.

Krueger, R. F., Hicks, B. M., & McGue, M. (2001). Altruism and antisocial behavior: Independent tendencies, unique personality correlates, distinct etiologies. *Psychological Science, 12,* 397–402.

Kuczynski, L., & De Mol, J. (2015). Dialectical models of socialization. In R. M. Lerner (Series Ed.) & W. F. Overton & P. C. M. Molenaar (Vol. Eds.), *Handbook of child psychology and developmental science: Vol. 1. Theory and method* (7th ed., pp. 323–368). Hoboken, NJ: Wiley.

Kuppens, S., Laurent, L., Heyvaert, M., & Onghena, P. (2013). Associations between parental psychological control and relational aggression in children and adolescents: A multilevel and sequential meta-analysis. *Developmental Psychology, 49,* 1697–1712.

Laible, D. (2004). Mother–child discourse surrounding a child's past behavior at 30 months: Links to emotional understanding and early conscience development at 36 months. *Merrill–Palmer Quarterly, 50,* 159–180.

Laible, D. (2011). Does it matter if preschool children and mothers discuss positive vs. negative events during reminiscing?: Links with mother-reported attachment, family emotional climate, and socioemotional development. *Social Development, 20,* 394–411.

Laible, D., & Murphy, T. P. (2014). Constructing moral, emotional, and relational understanding in the context of mother–child reminiscing. In C. Weinryb & H. Recchia (Eds.), *Talking about right and wrong: Parent–child conversations as contexts for moral development* (pp. 98–122). Cambridge, UK: Cambridge University Press.

Laible, D. J., Murphy, T. P., & Augustine, M. (2014). Adolescents' aggressive and prosocial behaviors: Links with social information processing, negative emotionality, moral affect, and moral cognition. *Journal of Genetic Psychology, 175*, 270–286.

Laible, D., & Panfile, T. (2009). Mother–child reminiscing in the context of secure attachment relationships. In J. Quas & R. Fivush (Eds.), *Emotion and memory in development: Biological, cognitive, and social considerations* (pp. 166–195). New York: Oxford University Press.

Laible, D., Panfile Murphy, T., & Augustine, M. (2013). Predicting the quality of mother–child reminiscing surrounding negative emotional events at 42 and 48 months old. *Journal of Cognition and Development, 14*, 270–291.

Laird, R. D., & Marrero, M. D. (2010). Information management and behavior problems: Is concealing misbehavior necessarily a sign of trouble? *Journal of Adolescence, 33*, 297–308.

Lamborn, S. D., Dornbusch, S. M., & Steinberg, L. (1996). Ethnicity and community context as moderators of the relations between family decision making and adolescent adjustment. *Child Development, 67*, 283–301.

Landry, S. H., Smith, K. E., & Swank, P. R. (2006). Responsive parenting: Establishing early foundations for social, communication, and independent problem-solving skills. *Developmental Psychology, 42*, 627–642.

Lansford, J. E., Chang, L., Dodge, K. A., Malone, P. S., Oburu, P., Palmérus, K., . . . Tapanya, S. (2005). Physical discipline and children's adjustment: Cultural normativeness as a moderator. *Child Development, 76*, 1234–1246.

Lansford, J. E., Deater-Deckard, K., Dodge, K. A., Bates, J. E., & Pettit, G. S. (2004). Ethnic differences in the link between physical discipline and later adolescent externalizing behaviors. *Journal of Child Psychology and Psychiatry, 45*, 801–812.

Lansford, J. E., Malone, P. S., Dodge, K. A., Chang, L., Chaudhary, N., Tapanya, S., . . . Deater-Deckard, K. (2010). Children's perceptions of maternal hostility as a mediator of the link between discipline and children's adjustment in four countries. *International Journal of Behavioral Development, 34*, 452–461.

Larson, R. W. (2001). How U.S. children and adolescents spend time: What it does (and doesn't) tell us about their development. *Current Directions in Psychological Science, 10*, 160–164.

Lay, K. L., Waters, E., & Park, K. A. (1989). Maternal responsiveness and child compliance: The role of mood as a mediator. *Child Development, 60*, 1405–1411.

Lee, K., Talwar, V., McCarthy, A., Ross, I., Evans, A., & Arruda, C. (2014). Can classic moral stories promote honesty in children? *Psychological Science, 25*, 1630–1636.

Lee, S. J., Grogan-Kaylor, A., & Berger, L. M. (2014). Parental spanking of 1-year-old children and subsequent child protective services involvement. *Child Abuse and Neglect, 38*, 875–883.

Leerkes, E. M., Blankson, A. N., & O'Brien, M. (2009). Differential effects of maternal sensitivity to infant distress and nondistress on social-emotional functioning. *Child Development, 80*, 762–775.

Leerkes, E. M., Weaver, J. M., & O'Brien, M. (2012). Differentiating maternal sensitivity to infant distress and non-distress. *Parenting: Science and Practice, 12*, 175–184.

Lengua, L. J. (2008). Anxiousness, frustration, and effortful control as moderators of the relation between parenting and adjustment in middle-childhood. *Social Development, 17*, 554–577.

Lepper, M. (1983). Social-control processes and the internalization of social values: An attributional perspective. In E. T. Higgins, D. Ruble, & W. W. Hartup (Eds.), *Social cognition and social development: A sociocultural perspective* (pp. 294–330). Cambridge, UK: Cambridge University Press.

Lepper, M. R., Greene, D., & Nisbett, R. E. (1973). Undermining children's intrinsic interest with extrinsic reward: A test of the "overjustification" hypothesis. *Journal of Personality and Social Psychology, 28*, 129–137.

Lewin, K., Lippitt, R., & White, R. K. (1939). Patterns of aggressive behavior in experimentally created "social climates." *Journal of Social Psychology, 10*, 269–299.

Lickel, B., Schmader, T., Curtis, M., Scarnier, M., & Ames, D. R. (2005). Vicarious shame and guilt. *Group Processes and Intergroup Relations, 8*, 145–157.

Lindsey, E. W., Cremeens, P. R., & Caldera, Y. M. (2010a). Mother–child and father–child mutuality in two contexts: Consequences for young children's peer relationships. *Infant and Child Development, 19*, 142–160.

Lindsey, E. W., Cremeens, P. R., & Caldera, Y. M. (2010b). Gender differences in mother–toddler and father–toddler verbal initiations and responses during a caregiving and play context. *Sex Roles, 63*, 399–411.

Lindsey, E. W., Cremeens, P. R., Colwell, M. J., & Caldera, Y. M. (2009). The structure of parent–child dyadic synchrony in toddlerhood and children's communication competence and self-control. *Social Development, 18*, 375–396.

Loeber, R., Green, S. M., Keenan, K., & Lahey, B. B. (1995). Which boys will fare worse?: Early predictors of the onset of conduct disorder in a six-year longitudinal study. *Journal of the American Academy of Child and Adolescent Psychiatry, 34*, 499–509.

Lorenz, K. A. (1970). Companions as factors in the bird's environment. In K. A. Lorenz, *Studies in animal and human behavior* (Vol. 1, pp. 101–254; R. Martin, Trans.). Cambridge, MA: Harvard University Press. (Original work published 1935)

Lundell, L. J., Grusec, J. E., McShane, K. E., & Davidov, M. (2008). Mother–adolescent conflict: Adolescent goals, maternal perspective-taking, and conflict intensity. *Journal of Research on Adolescence, 18*, 555–571.

Maccoby, E. E. (1983). Let's not overattribute to the attribution process: Comments on social cognition and behavior. In E. T. Higgins, D. N. Ruble, & W. W. Hartup (Eds.), *Social cognition and social development: A sociocultural perspective* (pp. 356–370). Cambridge, UK: Cambridge University Press.

Maccoby, E. E. (1992). The role of parents in the socialization of children: An historical overview. *Developmental Psychology, 28*, 1006–1017.

Maccoby, E. E. (2015). Historical overview of socialization research and theory. In J. E. Grusec & P. D. Hastings (Eds.), *Handbook of socialization: Theory and research* (2nd ed., pp. 3–32). New York: Guilford Press.

Maccoby, E. E., & Martin, J. A. (1983). Socialization in the context of the family: Parent–child interaction. In P. H. Mussen (Series Ed.) & E. M. Hetherington (Vol. Ed.), *Handbook of child psychology: Vol. 4. Socialization, personality, and social development* (4th ed., pp. 1–101). New York: Wiley.

MacDonald, K. (1992). Warmth as a developmental construct: An evolutionary analysis. *Child Development, 63*, 753–773.

Mageau, G. A., Sherman, A., Grusec, J. E., Koestner, R., & Bureau, J. S. (2017). Different ways of knowing a child and their relations to mother-reported autonomy support. *Social Development, 26*, 630–644.

Main, M., & Hesse, E. (1990). Parents' unresolved traumatic experiences are related to infant disorganized attachment status: Is frightened and/or frightening parental behavior the linking mechanism? In M. T. Greenberg, D. Cicchetti, & E. M. Cummings (Eds.), *Attachment in the preschool years: Theory, research, and intervention* (pp. 161–182). Chicago: University of Chicago Press.

Main, M., & Solomon, J. (1990). Procedures for identifying infants as disorganized/disoriented during the Ainsworth Strange Situation. In M. T. Greenberg, D. Cicchetti, & E. M. Cummings (Eds.), *Attachment in the preschool years: Theory, research, and intervention* (pp. 121–160). Chicago: University of Chicago Press.

Malti, T., Dys, S. P., Colasante, T., & Peplak, J. (2018). Emotions and morality: New developmental perspectives. In C. C. Helwig (Ed.), *New perspectives on moral development* (pp. 55–72). New York: Routledge.

Malti, T., & Krettenauer, T. (2013). The relation of moral emotion attributions to prosocial and antisocial behavior: A meta-analysis. *Child Development, 84*, 397–412.

Manongdo, J. A., & Ramírez García, J. I. (2011). Maternal parenting and mental health of Mexican American youth: A bidirectional and prospective approach. *Journal of Family Psychology, 25*, 261–270.

Markus, H. R., & Kitayama, S. (1991). Culture and the self: Implications for cognition, emotion, and motivation. *Psychological Review, 98*, 224–253.

Marshall, S. K., Tilton-Weaver, L. C., & Bosdet, L. (2005). Information management: Considering adolescents' regulation of parental knowledge. *Journal of Adolescence, 28*, 633–647.

Matas, L., Arend, R. A., & Sroufe, L. A. (1978). Continuity of adaptation in the second year: The relationship between quality of attachment and later competence. *Child Development, 49*, 547–556.

McDaniel, B. T., & Radesky, J. S. (2018). Technoference: Parent distraction with technology and associations with child behavior problems. *Child Development, 89*, 100–109.

McElwain, N. L., & Booth-LaForce, C. (2006). Maternal sensitivity to infant distress and nondistress as predictors of infant–mother attachment security. *Journal of Family Psychology, 20*, 247–255.

McLoyd, V. C., Kaplan, R., Hardaway, C. R., & Wood, D. (2007). Does endorsement of physical discipline matter?: Assessing moderating influences on the maternal and child psychological correlates of physical discipline in African American families. *Journal of Family Psychology, 21*, 165–175.

McLoyd, V. C., & Smith, J. (2002). Physical discipline and behavior problems in African American, European American, and Hispanic children: Emotional support as a moderator. *Journal of Marriage and Family, 64,* 40–53.

Meins, E., Fernyhough, C., Wainwright, R., Clark-Carter, D., Das Gupta, M., Fradley, E., & Tuckey, M. (2003). Pathways to understanding mind: Construct validity and predictive validity of maternal mind-mindedness. *Child Development, 74,* 1194–1211.

Meltzoff, A. N., & Moore, M. K. (1977). Imitation of facial and manual gestures by human neonates. *Science, 198,* 75–78.

Miller, J. G., & Bersoff, D. M. (1992). Culture and moral judgment: How are conflicts between justice and interpersonal responsibilities resolved? *Journal of Personality and Social Psychology, 62,* 541–554.

Miller, J. G., & Bersoff, D. M. (1994). Cultural influences on the moral status of reciprocity and the discounting of endogenous motivation. *Personality and Social Psychology Bulletin, 20,* 592–602.

Miller, P. J. (1994). Narrative practices: Their role in socialization and self-construction. In U. Neisser & R. Fivush (Eds.), *The remembering self: Accuracy and construction in the self-narrative* (pp. 158–179). New York: Cambridge University Press.

Miller, P. J., Fung, H., Lin, S., Chen, E. C. H., & Boldt, B. R. (2012). How socialization happens on the ground: Narrative practices as alternate socializing pathways in Taiwanese and European-American families. *Monographs of the Society for Research in Child Development, 77*(1), 1–140.

Miller, R. L., Brickman, P., & Bolen, D. (1975). Attribution versus persuasion as a means for modifying behavior. *Journal of Personality and Social Psychology, 31,* 430–441.

Morris, A. S., Silk, J. S., Morris, M. D., Steinberg, L., Aucoin, K. J., & Keyes, A. W. (2011). The influence of mother–child emotion regulation strategies on children's expression of anger and sadness. *Developmental Psychology, 47,* 213–225.

Morris, A. S., Silk, J. S., Steinberg, L., Terranova, A. M., & Kithakye, M. (2010). Concurrent and longitudinal links between children's externalizing behavior in school and observed anger regulation in the mother–child dyad. *Journal of Psychopathology and Behavioral Assessment, 32,* 48–56.

Morton, J. B., & Trehub, S. E. (2001). Children's understanding of emotion in speech. *Child Development, 72,* 834–843.

Ng, F. F.-Y., Kenney-Benson, G. A., & Pomerantz, E. M. (2004). Children's achievement moderates the effects of mothers' use of control and autonomy support. *Child Development, 75,* 764–780.

Nucci, L. (1984). Evaluating teachers as social agents: Students' ratings of domain appropriate and domain inappropriate teacher responses to transgression. *American Educational Research Journal, 21,* 367–378.

Oldershaw, L. (2002). *A national survey of parents of young children: Executive summary.* Toronto, ON: Invest in Kids.

O'Neal, E. E., & Plumert, J. M. (2014). Mother–child conversations about safety:

Implications for socializing safety values in children. *Journal of Pediatric Psychology, 39,* 481–491.

Oppenheim, D., Sagi, A., & Lamb, M. E. (1988). Infant–adult attachments on the kibbutz and their relation to socioemotional development 4 years later. *Developmental Psychology, 24,* 427–433.

Oppliger, P. A. (2007). Effects of gender stereotyping on socialization. In R. W. Preiss, B. M. Gayle, N. Burrell, M. Allen, & J. Bryant (Eds.), *Mass media effects research: Advances through meta-analysis* (pp. 199–214). New York: Routledge.

Ottoni-Wilhelm, M., Estell, D. B., & Perdue, N. H. (2014). Role-modeling and conversations about giving in the socialization of adolescent charitable giving and volunteering. *Journal of Adolescence, 37,* 53–66.

Padilla-Walker, L. M. (2007). Characteristics of mother–child interactions related to adolescents' positive values and behaviors. *Journal of Marriage and Family, 69,* 675–686.

Padilla-Walker, L. M. (2008). "My mom makes me so angry!": Adolescent perceptions of mother–child interactions as correlates of adolescent emotions. *Social Development, 17,* 306–325.

Padilla-Walker, L. M., & Carlo, G. (2004). "It's not fair!": Adolescents' constructions of appropriateness of parental reactions. *Journal of Youth and Adolescence, 33,* 389–401.

Padilla-Walker, L. M., & Thompson, R. A. (2005). Combating conflicting messages of values: A closer look at parental strategies. *Social Development, 14,* 305–323.

Parpal, M., & Maccoby, E. E. (1985). Maternal responsiveness and subsequent child compliance. *Child Development, 56,* 1326–1334.

Patterson, G. R. (1980). Mothers: The unacknowledged victims. *Monographs of the Society for Research in Child Development, 45*(5), 1–54.

Patterson, G. R. (1997). Performance models for parenting: A social interactional perspective. In J. E. Grusec & L. Kuczynski (Eds.), *Parenting and children's internalization of values: A handbook of contemporary theory* (pp. 193–226). New York: Wiley.

Peterson, L. (1982). Altruism and the development of internal control: An integrative model. *Merrill–Palmer Quarterly, 22,* 197–222.

Pettit, G. S., Bates, J. E., & Dodge, K. A. (1997). Supportive parenting, ecological context, and children's adjustment: A seven-year longitudinal study. *Child Development, 68,* 908–923.

Piaget, J. (1932). *Le jugement moral chez l'enfant [The moral judgment of the child].* Paris: Alcan.

Piaget, J. (1936). *The origin of intelligence in the child.* London: Routledge & Kegan Paul.

Prot, S., Anderson, C. A., Gentile, D. A., Warburton, W., Saleem, M., Groves, C. L., & Brown, S. C. (2015). Media as agents of socialization. In J. E. Grusec & P. D. Hastings (Eds.), *Handbook of socialization: Theory and research* (2nd ed., pp. 276–300). New York: Guilford Press.

Pulfrey, C., & Butera, F. (2013). Why neoliberal values of self-enhancement lead to cheating in higher education: A motivational account. *Psychological Science, 24*, 2153–2162.

Puntambekar, S., & Hubscher, R. (2005). Tools for scaffolding students in a complex learning environment: What have we gained and what have we missed? *Educational Psychologist, 40*, 1–12.

Raikes, H. A., & Thompson, R. A. (2008). Attachment security and parenting quality predict children's problem-solving, attributions, and loneliness with peers. *Attachment and Human Development, 10*, 319–344.

Raikes, H. A., Virmani, E. A., Thompson, R. A., & Hatton, H. (2013). Declines in peer conflict from preschool through first grade: Influences from early attachment and social information processing. *Attachment and Human Development, 15*, 65–82.

Reese, E., & Fivush, R. (1993). Parental styles of talking about the past. *Developmental Psychology, 29*, 596–606.

Reese, E., Haden, C. A., & Fivush, R. (1993). Mother–child conversations about the past: Relationships of style and memory over time. *Cognitive Development, 8*, 403–430.

Reese, E., & Newcombe, R. (2007). Training mothers in elaborative reminiscing enhances children's autobiographical memory and narrative. *Child Development, 78*, 1153–1170.

Robertson, J. (1953). *A two-year-old goes to hospital* [Film]. London: Tavistock Child Development Research Unit. (Available through the Penn State Audiovisual Services, University Park, PA)

Robertson, J. (1969). *John, 17 months* [Film]. New York: New York University Film Library.

Rogoff, B., Moore, L., Correa-Chávez, M., & Dexter, A. (2015). Children develop cultural repertoires through engaging in everyday routines and practices. In J. E. Grusec & P. D. Hastings (Eds.), *Handbook of socialization: Theory and research* (2nd ed., pp. 472–498). New York: Guilford Press.

Rohner, R. P., & Britner, P. A. (2002). Worldwide mental health correlates of parental acceptance–rejection: Review of cross-cultural and intracultural evidence. *Cross-Cultural Research, 36*, 16–47.

Rossano, M. J. (2012). The essential role of ritual in the transmission and reinforcement of social norms. *Psychological Bulletin, 138*, 529–549.

Roth, G. (2008). Perceived parental conditional regard and autonomy support as predictors of young adults' self- versus other-oriented prosocial tendencies. *Journal of Personality, 76*, 513–534.

Roth, G., Assor, A., Niemiec, C. P., Ryan, R. M., & Deci, E. L. (2009). The emotional and academic consequences of parental conditional regard: Comparing conditional positive regard, conditional negative regard, and autonomy support as parenting practices. *Developmental Psychology, 45*, 1119–1142.

Roth-Hanania, R., Davidov, M., & Zahn-Waxler, C. (2011). Empathy development from 8 to 16 months: Early signs of concern for others. *Infant Behavior and Development, 34*, 447–458.

Rothbaum, F., & Trommsdorff, G. (2007). Do roots and wings complement or oppose one another?: The socialization of relatedness and autonomy in cultural context. In J. E. Grusec & P. D. Hastings (Eds.), *Handbook of socialization: Theory and research* (pp. 461–489). New York: Guilford Press.

Rothbaum, F., & Weisz, J. R. (1994). Parental caregiving and child externalizing behavior in nonclinical samples: A meta-analysis. *Psychological Bulletin, 116,* 55–74.

Rothbaum, F., Weisz, J., Pott, M., Miyake, K., & Morelli, G. (2000). Attachment and culture: Security in the United States and Japan. *American Psychologist, 55,* 1093–1104.

Rubin, K. H., Burgess, K. B., & Hastings, P. D. (2002). Stability and social-behavioral consequences of toddlers' inhibited temperament and parenting behaviors. *Child Development, 73,* 483–495.

Rudy, D., & Grusec, J. E. (2001). Correlates of authoritarian parenting in individualist and collectivist cultures and implications for understanding the transmission of values. *Journal of Cross-Cultural Psychology, 32,* 202–212.

Rudy, D., & Grusec, J. E. (2006). Authoritarian parenting in individualist and collectivist groups: Associations with maternal emotion and cognition and children's self-esteem. *Journal of Family Psychology, 20,* 68–78.

Ryan, R. M., & Deci, E. L. (2000). Self-determination theory and the facilitation of intrinsic motivation, social development, and well-being. *American Psychologist, 55,* 68–78.

Ryan, R. M., & Deci, E. L. (2017). *Self-determination theory: Basic psychological needs in motivation, development, and wellness.* New York: Guilford Press.

Sabbagh, M. A., & Callanan, M. A. (1998). Metarepresentation in action: 3-, 4-, and 5-year-olds' developing theories of mind in parent–child conversations. *Developmental Psychology, 34,* 491–502.

Schaffer, H. R., & Crook, C. K. (1980). Child compliance and maternal control techniques. *Developmental Psychology, 16,* 54–61.

Schmidt, M. F., Rakoczy, H., & Tomasello, M. (2011). Young children attribute normativity to novel actions without pedagogy or normative language. *Developmental Science, 14,* 530–539.

Schneider, B. H., Atkinson, L., & Tardif, C. (2001). Child–parent attachment and children's peer relations: A quantitative review. *Developmental Psychology, 37,* 86–100.

Schwartz, S. H. (1992). Universals in the content and structure of values: Theoretical advances and empirical tests in 20 countries. In M. P. Zanna (Ed.), *Advances in experimental social psychology* (Vol. 25, pp. 1–65). San Diego, CA: Academic Press.

Schwartz, S. H., & Bardi, A. (2001). Value hierarchies across cultures: Taking a similarities perspective. *Journal of Cross-Cultural Psychology, 32,* 268–290.

Schwartz, S. H., Cieciuch, J., Vecchione, M., Davidov, E., Fischer, R., Beierlein, C., . . . Konty, M. (2012). Refining the theory of basic individual values. *Journal of Personality and Social Psychology, 103,* 663–688.

Sears, R. R., Maccoby, E. E., & Levin, H. (1957). *Patterns of child rearing.* Evanston, IL: Row, Peterson.

Sears, R. R., Whiting, J. W. M., Nowlis, V., & Sears, P. S. (1953). Some child-rearing antecedents of aggression and dependency in young children. *Genetic Psychology Monographs, 47*, 135–236.

Seay, B., & Harlow, H. F. (1965). Maternal separation in the rhesus monkey. *Journal of Nervous and Mental Disease, 140*, 434–441.

Sherif, M., & Sherif, C. W. (1953). *Groups in harmony and tension.* New York: Harper.

Sherman, A., Grusec, J. E., & Almas, A. N. (2017). Mothers' knowledge of what reduces distress in their adolescents: Impact on the development of adolescent approach coping. *Parenting: Science and Practice, 17*, 187–199.

Siegal, M., & Barclay, M. S. (1985). Children's evaluations of fathers' socialization behavior. *Developmental Psychology, 21*, 1090–1096.

Siegal, M., & Cowen, J. (1984). Appraisals of intervention: The mother's versus the culprit's behavior as determinants of children's evaluations of discipline techniques. *Child Development, 55*, 1760–1766.

Simmel, G. (1902). The number of members as determining the sociological form of the group. *American Journal of Sociology, 8*, 1–46.

Simons, R. L., Wu, C. I., Lin, K. H., Gordon, L., & Conger, R. D. (2000). A cross-cultural examination of the link between corporal punishment and adolescent antisocial behavior. *Criminology, 38*, 47–80.

Smetana, J. G. (1981). Preschool children's conceptions of moral and social rules. *Child Development, 52*, 1333–1336.

Smetana, J. G. (1988). Concepts of self and social convention: Adolescents' and parents' reasoning about hypothetical and actual family conflicts. In M. R. Gunnar & W. A. Collins (Eds.), *Minnesota Symposia on Child Psychology: Vol. 21. Development during the transition to adolescence* (pp. 79–122). Hillsdale, NJ: Erlbaum.

Smetana, J. G. (1997). Parenting and the development of social knowledge reconceptualized: A social domain analysis. In J. E. Grusec & L. Kuczynski (Eds.), *Parenting and children's internalization of values: A handbook of contemporary theory* (pp. 162–192). New York: Wiley.

Smetana, J. G. (2011). *Adolescents, families, and social development: How teens construct their worlds.* Chichester, UK: Wiley.

Smetana, J. G., Metzger, A., Gettman, D. C., & Campione-Barr, N. (2006). Disclosure and secrecy in adolescent–parent relationships. *Child Development, 77*, 201–217.

Smetana, J. G., Robinson, J., & Rote, W. M. (2015). Socialization in adolescence. In J. E. Grusec & P. D. Hastings (Eds.), *Handbook of socialization: Theory and research* (2nd ed., pp. 60–84). New York: Guilford Press.

Smetana, J. G., Villalobos, M., Tasopoulos-Chan, M., Gettman, D. C., & Campione-Barr, N. (2009). Early and middle adolescents' disclosure to parents about activities in different domains. *Journal of Adolescence, 32*, 693–713.

Smith, T. W., Marsden, P., Hout, M., & Kim, J. (2013). *General social surveys, 1972–2012* [Machine-readable data file]. Chicago: National Opinion Research Center [Producer], Storrs, CT: Roper Center for Public Opinion Research, University of Connecticut [Distributor].

Snyder, J., Reid, J., & Patterson, G. (2003). A social learning model of child and adolescent antisocial behavior. In B. B. Lahey, T. E. Moffitt, & A. Caspi (Eds.), *Causes of conduct disorder and juvenile delinquency* (pp. 27–48). New York: Guilford Press.

Soenens, B., Vansteenkiste, M., Luyckx, K., & Goossens, L. (2006). Parenting and adolescent problem behavior: An integrated model with adolescent self-disclosure and perceived parental knowledge as intervening variables. *Developmental Psychology, 42*, 305–318.

Sorce, J. F., & Emde, R. N. (1981). Mother's presence is not enough: Effect of emotional availability on infant exploration. *Developmental Psychology, 17*, 737–745.

Spagnola, M., & Fiese, B. H. (2007). Family routines and rituals: A context for development in the lives of young children. *Infants and Young Children, 20*, 284–299.

Spruit, A., van Vugt, E., van der Put, C., van der Stouwe, T., & Stams, G. J. (2016). Sports participation and juvenile delinquency: A meta-analytic review. *Journal of Youth and Adolescence, 45*, 655–671.

Sroufe, L. A., & Waters, E. (1977). Attachment as an organizational construct. *Child Development, 48*, 1184–1199.

Stattin, H., & Kerr, M. (2000). Parental monitoring: A reinterpretation. *Child Development, 71*, 1072–1085.

Staub, E. (1979). *Positive prosocial behavior and morality.* New York: Academic Press.

Stayton, D. J., Hogan, R., & Ainsworth, M. D. S. (1971). Infant obedience and maternal behavior: The origins of socialization reconsidered. *Child Development, 42*, 1057–1069.

Strassberg, Z., Dodge, K. A., Pettit, G. S., & Bates, J. E. (1994). Spanking in the home and children's subsequent aggression toward kindergarten peers. *Development and Psychopathology, 6*, 445–461.

Straus, M. A. (1996). Spanking and the making of a violent society. *Pediatrics, 98*, 837–842.

Taheri, S. A., & Welsh, B. C. (2016). After-school programs for delinquency prevention: A systematic review and meta-analysis. *Youth Violence and Juvenile Justice, 14*, 272–290.

Takahashi, K. (1986). Examining the Strange-Situation procedure with Japanese mothers and 12-month-old infants. *Developmental Psychology, 22*, 265–270.

Talwar, V., Yachison, S., & Leduc, K. (2016). Promoting honesty: The influence of stories on children's lie-telling behaviors and moral understanding. *Infant and Child Development, 25*, 484–501.

Taylor, J. H., & Walker, L. J. (1997). Moral climate and the development of moral reasoning: The effects of dyadic discussions between young offenders. *Journal of Moral Education, 26*, 21–43.

Thapar, A., Rice, F., Hay, D., Boivin, J., Langley, K., Van Den Bree, M., . . . Harold, G. (2009). Prenatal smoking might not cause attention-deficit/hyperactivity disorder: Evidence from a novel design. *Biological Psychiatry, 66*, 722–727.

Thompson, R. A. (2006). The development of the person: Social understanding, relationships, self, conscience. In W. Damon & R. M. Lerner (Series Eds.) & N. Eisenberg (Vol. Ed.), *Handbook of child psychology: Vol. 3. Social, emotional, and personality development* (6th ed., pp. 24–98). Hoboken, NJ: Wiley.

Thompson, R. A. (2016). Early attachment and later development: Reframing the questions. In J. Cassidy & P. R. Shaver (Eds.), *Handbook of attachment: Theory, research, and clinical applications* (3rd ed., pp. 330–348). New York: Guilford Press.

Tildesley, E. A., & Andrews, J. A. (2008). The development of children's intentions to use alcohol: Direct and indirect effects of parent alcohol use and parenting behaviors. *Psychology of Addictive Behaviors, 22,* 326–339.

Tizard, B., & Hughes, M. (2002). *Young children learning.* Oxford, UK: Wiley-Blackwell.

Tokić, A., & Pećnik, N. (2011). Parental behaviors related to adolescents' self-disclosure: Adolescents' views. *Journal of Social and Personal Relationships, 28,* 201–222.

Trevarthen, C., Kokkinaki, T., & Fiamenghi, G. A., Jr. (1999). What infants' imitations communicate: With mothers, with fathers and with peers. In J. Nadel & G. Butterworth (Eds.), *Cambridge studies in cognitive perceptual development: Imitation in infancy* (pp. 127–185). New York: Cambridge University Press.

Trickett, P. K., & Kuczynski, L. (1986). Children's misbehaviors and parental discipline strategies in abusive and nonabusive families. *Developmental Psychology, 22,* 115–123.

Tronick, E., Als, H., Adamson, L., Wise, S., & Brazelton, T. B. (1978). The infant's response to entrapment between contradictory messages in face-to-face interaction. *Journal of the American Academy of Child Psychiatry, 17,* 1–13.

Turiel, E. (1983). *The development of social knowledge: Morality and convention.* New York: Cambridge University Press.

Turiel, E. (2018). Reasoning at the root of morality. In K. Gray & J. Graham (Eds.), *Atlas of moral psychology* (pp. 9–19). New York: Guilford Press.

Turner, V. D., & Berkowitz, M. W. (2005). Scaffolding morality: Positioning a socio-cultural construct. *New Ideas in Psychology, 23,* 174–184.

Underwood, B., Froming, W. J., & Moore, B. S. (1977). Mood, attention, and altruism: A search for mediating variables. *Developmental Psychology, 13,* 541–542.

Uzefovsky, F., Döring, A. K., & Knafo-Noam, A. (2016). Values in middle childhood: Social and genetic contributions. *Social Development, 25,* 482–502.

Vaish, A., & Tomasello, M. (2014). The early ontogeny of human cooperation and morality. In M. Killen & J. G. Smetana (Eds.), *Handbook of moral development* (pp. 279–298). New York: Psychology Press.

Van Bergen, P. V., Salmon, K., Dadds, M. R., & Allen, J. (2009). The effects of mother training in emotion-rich, elaborative reminiscing on children's shared recall and emotion knowledge. *Journal of Cognition and Development, 10,* 162–187.

Van de Vondervoort, J. W., & Hamlin, J. K. (2016). Evidence for intuitive moral-ity: Preverbal infants make sociomoral evaluations. *Child Development Per-spectives, 10,* 143–148.

van Goethem, A., van Hoof, A., Orobio de Castro, B., Van Aken, M., & Hart, D. (2014). The role of reflection in the effects of community service on adolescent development: A meta-analysis. *Child Development, 85,* 2114–2130.

van IJzendoorn, M. H., & Sagi-Schwartz, A. (2008). Cross-cultural patterns of attachment: Universal and contextual dimensions. In J. Cassidy & P. R. Shaver (Eds.), *Handbook of attachment: Theory, research, and clinical applications* (2nd ed., pp. 880–905). New York: Guilford Press.

Van Petegem, S., Soenens, B., Vansteenkiste, M., & Beyers, W. (2015). Rebels with a cause?: Adolescent defiance from the perspective of reactance theory and self-determination theory. *Child Development, 86,* 903–918.

Vecchione, M., Döring, A. K., Alessandri, G., Marsicano, G., & Bardi, A. (2016). Reciprocal relations across time between basic values and value-expressive behaviors: A longitudinal study among children. *Social Development, 25,* 528–547.

Verhage, M. L., Schuengel, C., Madigan, S., Fearon, R. M., Oosterman, M., Cassibba, R., . . . van IJzendoorn, M. H. (2016). Narrowing the transmis-sion gap: A synthesis of three decades of research on intergenerational trans-mission of attachment. *Psychological Bulletin, 142,* 337–366.

Vinik, J. (2013). *Children's acquisition of values within the family: Domains of socializa-tion assessed with autobiographical narratives.* Unpublished doctoral dissertation, University of Toronto, Toronto, ON, Canada.

Vinik, J., Almas, A., & Grusec, J. (2011). Mothers' knowledge of what distresses and what comforts their children predicts children's coping, empathy, and prosocial behavior. *Parenting: Science and Practice, 11,* 56–71.

Vinik, J., Johnston, M., Grusec, J. E., & Farrell, R. (2013). Understanding the learning of values using a domains-of-socialization framework. *Journal of Moral Education, 42,* 475–493.

Vuchinich, S., Emery, R. E., & Cassidy, J. (1988). Family members and third parties in dyadic family conflict: Strategies, alliances, and outcomes. *Child Development, 59,* 1293–1302.

Vygotsky, L. S. (1978). *Minds in society.* Cambridge, MA: Harvard University Press.

Wainryb, C., & Recchia, H. (2014). Parent–child conversations as contexts for moral development. In C. Wainryb & H. Recchia (Eds.), *Talking about right and wrong: Parent–child conversations as contexts for moral development* (pp. 3–18). Cambridge, UK: Cambridge University Press.

Waizenhofer, R. N., Buchanan, C. M., & Jackson-Newsom, J. (2004). Mothers' and fathers' knowledge of adolescents' daily activities: Its sources and its links with adolescent adjustment. *Journal of Family Psychology, 18,* 348–360.

Walker, L. J., Hennig, K. H., & Krettenauer, T. (2000). Parent and peer con-texts for children's moral reasoning development. *Child Development, 71,* 1033–1048.

Walters, R. H., & Parke, R. D. (1964). Social motivation, dependency, and susceptibility to social influence. In L. Berkowitz (Ed.), *Advances in experimental social psychology* (Vol. 1, pp. 231–276). New York: Academic Press.

Walton, K., Kuczynski, L., Haycraft, E., Breen, A., & Haines, J. (2017). Time to re-think picky eating?: A relational approach to understanding picky eating. *International Journal of Behavioral Nutrition and Physical Activity, 14*, 62.

Wang, M. T., & Huguley, J. P. (2012). Parental racial socialization as a moderator of the effects of racial discrimination on educational success among African American adolescents. *Child Development, 83*, 1716–1731.

Weiner, B. (Ed.). (1974). *Achievement motivation and attribution theory.* Morristown, NJ: General Learning Press.

Weinfield, N. S., Sroufe, L. A., Egeland, B., & Carlson, E. (2008). Individual differences in infant–caregiver attachment: Conceptual and empirical aspects of security. In J. Cassidy & P. R. Shaver (Eds.), *Handbook of attachment: Theory, research, and clinical applications* (2nd ed., pp. 78–101). New York: Guilford Press.

Wills, T. A., Sargent, J. D., Gibbons, F. X., Gerrard, M., & Stoolmiller, M. (2009). Movie exposure to alcohol cues and adolescent alcohol problems: A longitudinal analysis in a national sample. *Psychology of Addictive Behaviors, 23*, 23–35.

Winnicott, D. W. (1953). Psychoses and child care. *Psychology and Psychotherapy: Theory, Research and Practice, 26*, 68–74.

Wismer Fries, A. B., Shirtcliff, E. A., & Pollak, S. D. (2008). Neuroendocrine dysregulation following early social deprivation in children. *Developmental Psychobiology, 50*, 588–599.

Wood, D., Bruner, J. S., & Ross, G. (1976). The role of tutoring in problem solving. *Journal of Child Psychology and Psychiatry, 17*, 89–100.

Wood, D., & Middleton, D. (1975). A study of assisted problem-solving. *British Journal of Psychology, 66*, 181–191.

World Health Organization. (2002). Child abuse and neglect by parents and caregivers. In World Health Organization, *World report on violence and health* (pp. 59–86). Geneva, Switzerland: Author.

Wynn, K., & Bloom, P. (2014). The moral baby. In M. Killen & J. G. Smetana (Eds.), *Handbook of moral development* (2nd ed., pp. 435–453). New York: Psychology Press.

Yan, N., & Dix, T. (2014). Mothers' early depressive symptoms and children's first-grade adjustment: A transactional analysis of child withdrawal as a mediator. *Journal of Child Psychology and Psychiatry, 55*, 495–504.

Ybarra, M. L., Mitchell, K. J., Hamburger, M., Diener-West, M., & Leaf, P. J. (2011). X-rated material and perpetration of sexually aggressive behavior among children and adolescents: Is there a link? *Aggressive Behavior, 37*, 1–18.

Youniss, J. (1980). *Parents and peers in social development: A Sullivan–Piaget perspective.* Chicago: University of Chicago Press.

Zaman, W., & Fivush, R. (2013). Gender differences in elaborative parent–child emotion and play narratives. *Sex Roles, 68*, 591–604.

# Index

Note. *f* or *t* following a page number indicates a figure or a table.